G
Health
& Great
Sex
After 40

A
Woman's
Guide

———

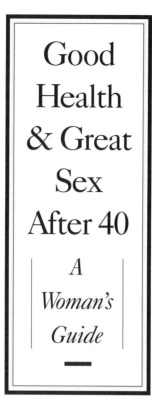

Good Health & Great Sex After 40

A *Woman's Guide*

MORTON A. STENCHEVER, M.D.
Professor and Chairman Emeritus of Obstetrics and Gynecology
University of Washington School of Medicine
Seattle, Washington

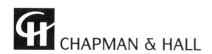

CHAPMAN & HALL

I (T)P® **International Thomson Publishing**
Thomson Science

New York • Albany • Bonn • Boston • Cincinnati • Detroit • London • Madrid • Melbourne
Mexico City • Pacific Grove • Paris • San Francisco • Singapore • Tokyo • Toronto • Washington

Cover design: Trudi Gershenov
Cover photo: © 1997 Comstock, Inc.
Copyright© 1997 Chapman & Hall

Printed in the United States of America

For more information, contact:

Chapman & Hall
115 Fifth Avenue
New York, NY 10003

Chapman & Hall
2-6 Boundary Row
London SE1 8HN
England

Thomas Nelson Australia
102 Dodds Street
South Melbourne, 3205
Victoria, Australia

Chapman & Hall GmbH
Postfach 100 263
D-69442 Weinheim
Germany

International Thomson Editores
Campos Eliseos 385, Piso 7
Col. Polanco
11560 Mexico D. F.
Mexico

International Thomson Publishing - Japan
Hirakawacho-cho Kyowa Building, 3F
1-2-1 Hirakawacho-cho
Chiyoda-ku, 102 Tokyo
Japan

International Thomson Publishing Asia
221 Henderson Road #05-10
Henderson Building
Singapore 0315

1 2 3 4 5 6 7 8 9 10 XXX 01 00 99 98 97
Library of Congress Cataloging-in-Publication Data

Good Health & Great Sex After 40: A Woman's Guide
Morton A. Stenchever.
p. cm.
Includes index.
ISBN 0-412-12681-8 (alk. paper)
1. Middle aged women—Health and hygiene. 2. Aged women—Health and hygiene. I. Stenchever, Morton A.
RA778.G696 1997
613'.04244--dc21

97-11504
CIP

British Library Cataloguing in Pubication Data available

To order this or any other Chapman & Hall book, please contact **International Thomson Publishing, 7625 Empire Drive, Florence, KY 41042.** Phone: (606) 525-6600 or 1-800-842-3636. Fax: (606) 525-7778. e-mail: order@chaphall.com.

For a complete listing of Chapman & Hall's titles, send your request to **Chapman & Hall, Dept. BC, 115 Fifth Avenue, New York, NY 10003.**

To my patients who stimulated my interest and inspired me to write this book and to my wife, Diane, for her insights and critical review

Table of Contents

Preface

In 1900, the average American woman's life expectancy was just under fifty years. Today the average age of a woman at menopause is just over fifty years. Thus, a century ago, the average woman did not live long enough to reach menopause. The problems related to aging were the concern of only a very few. Currently, life expectancy for a woman in the United States is 79.1 years, and it is estimated that it will be well past eighty by the turn of the century. Biologists feel that a reasonable life expectancy for a human is eighty-five years. Certainly, many live well past this age. There are many reasons that women live longer today than they did one-hundred years ago. Many of these will be touched upon in this book. Of greater importance, however, this book will address the ways in which women can develop healthy practices, prevent disease, and maintain a healthy emotional state, thereby preventing deterioration for as long as possible—it is to be hoped, to just before death. This is in contrast to the slow decline that many women formerly suffered from the time of their middle age. It is possible to achieve such goals, but to do so requires the cooperation of each woman and her health care providers.

Currently, 9.5 percent of the women in the United States are over the age of sixty. By the year 2025, 12.5 percent of women will be past this age. It is not only important for women to maintain good health and productivity, but it is also important for society in general that they do so in order to avoid a major economic and social disaster.

In 1996, I edited and published *Health Care for the Older Woman,* which was written for the use of doctors and was carefully referenced. The present book does not include references, since I intended it to be used by the general public and wished it to be easily understandable. Those of you who wish to find specific references may do so by consulting the more technical book which had several expert contributors.

There is now a great deal of scientific information available to help women prolong their vitality, good health, and a good outlook, as well as to prolong life itself.

There is also a great deal of misinformation in the public domain. By citing typical cases and by offering analyses of current information, I will try to help you develop a lifestyle that will work for you to maintain good health and a good quality of life for as long as possible.

MORTON A. STENCHEVER, M.D.

CHAPTER 1

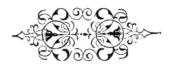

The Aging Process:
How to Live with It and How to Fight It

Growing old is not bad! You *can* maintain your health and vitality! You *can* maintain your attractiveness. And you *can* grow emotionally and intellectually. Your experiences have given you a good basis for this development, and the decrease in demands on your time that often occurs in later life can give you the opportunity. Usually you are in control of your fate and have the power to greatly influence the direction that you take. Your positive attitude will strongly help to make all this possible.

Let me illustrate with a tale of two women, both seventy-six years old. The first, Wendy, became a patient of mine when she was sixty years old. Although she suffered from hypertension and was taking antihypertensive drugs, she was thin, blond, and perky, appearing to be about forty-five years old. She led (and continues to lead) an active life, playing tennis three times a week and belonging to a bridge group and two book clubs. Her husband, who is ten years her senior, still runs his own business, and the couple vacations for two weeks in the south in winter and usually travels to distant places for two or three weeks each summer. Now, at seventy-six, Wendy maintains the same pace and still looks fifteen years younger than her age, and she and her husband still maintain a satisfying sex life. Although she has had a few illnesses and has required surgery on a foot and a shoulder, she still has the positive outlook she has always enjoyed. She takes care of herself, her clothes are stylish, her hair is cut short and colored, and her makeup is properly understated. She accentuates the positive.

Lila, on the other hand, is also seventy-six, and she has been a patient of mine since she was sixty-two. She is a retired businesswoman and has no financial problems. She cared for her elderly father until he died four years ago. Over the years, she has become less active than before. She does not socialize with friends and, although she has been widowed for twenty years, has not pursued any relationships with men, even though she had some opportunities several years ago. Over the past fifteen years she has gained fifty pounds in spite of attempts to try to improve her diet. She has had both knees replaced because of arthritis and has arthritis in several other joints. Because of her discomfort, she has become more and more inactive, and with this she has become depressed. She sees multiple physicians for multiple complaints and is not a happy woman.

The contrast between these two women is obviously striking, but many of their differences were due to decisions they made along the way.

Until very recently, the years from middle age to old age were characterized for most people by a fairly steep slide in health and physical abilities. Since middle age for women encompasses the time of menopause, this point, usually around age fifty, represented for many the beginning of the descent. Today, a better understanding of ways to maintain good health and utilize the advances of medical science has made it possible to extend the time when a woman's health begins to decline until well into old age. To accomplish this, the woman should, of course, be given the benefit of modern medical care so that acute and chronic illnesses can be diagnosed and managed early in order to effect a cure or at least to blunt the effects of a chronic condition. Much of this book will be devoted to defining these specific problems and discussing how a woman can obtain health care should she be afflicted by any of them. On the other hand, maintaining good health and fitness is something you can usually do for yourself. This chapter outlines healthy practices that you can begin today and that should not only improve your health and longevity but also make you feel good. (See Table 1.1.)

TABLE 1.1.   Health Practices That You Should Undertake

Good nutrition

Adequate sleep

Proper exercise

Hormone replacement therapy

Smoking cessation

Limiting alcohol use

Using medications appropriately

Using seat belts and helmets

Wearing safe footwear

Moving with caution

Avoiding inappropriate and strenuous tasks and activities

Using firearms safely

DIETARY HABITS AND NUTRITION

Good dietary habits are closely related to good health, but maintaining good dietary habits, as most of us know, is difficult. To some extent nature works against us. After age fifty, caloric requirements decrease because of a change in general metabolism. Thus, the tendency of the body is to save more from less. Part of the problem may also be that after age fifty a woman may not be quite as active as she was before, so that the opportunity to burn off calories is decreased. In general, women past the age of fifty rarely require more than 1,700 calories a day to maintain their weight. Increases in calories above this will generally increase fat deposits, particularly in the breasts, abdomen, and thighs.

CASE STUDY

Doris is a fifty-three-year-old attractive woman who has always been somewhat overweight. When she consulted me for her annual health checkup, she carried 175 pounds on her five-foot, four-inch frame. She is a homemaker and mother of three grown children, all of whom have left home. She lives with her husband, a successful attorney, and is active with clubs and volunteer work. She states that through her thirties and forties she was able to wear a size 12 dress and maintained her weight at about 140 pounds. This required frequent dieting, and over the years she tried many different diet plans, including liquid diets, Weight Watchers, and fad diets that were popular at the time. She was always able to lose ten to fifteen pounds and could frequently keep them off for six to eight months. Inevitably, the weight would return, usually with a dividend of a few extra pounds. During those years she was very busy with her children's activities as well as her own. When she was fifty years old, she had an acute gall bladder attack and had to have her gall bladder removed. At that time she weighed 155 pounds. During that year she went through menopause and decided not to take hormone replacement therapy. Her health continued to be quite good, but her weight continued to rise, and she has gained twenty more pounds during the past three years. She feels reasonably well but does not seem to have the energy she had in the past, which has led to her becoming less active. She has developed some arthritis in her knees for which a nonsteroidal anti-inflammatory drug, ibuprofen, has been prescribed. She is quite dismayed by the fact that she now wears a size 16 dress.

Doris is a very typical case. She has always had a tendency to gain weight, but she has managed this with crash or fad diets from time to time, motivated by her wish to look slim and to fit into her size 12 dresses. During her thirties and forties she was extremely active and was able to burn off many of the calories that she accumulated in her diet. The frequent fluctuations in her weight probably contributed to her gall bladder disease and led to the necessity for the removal of her gall bladder. After menopause, when her metabolic needs became even less, she also experienced a decrease in activity due to the change in her life circumstances at that time. As her weight increased she developed some signs and symptoms of arthritis in her knees, and this further decreased her activities and her ability to burn off calories. All of this contributed to a steady weight gain. A nutritionist working with me placed Doris on a well-balanced 1,500-calorie diet. She also encouraged her to begin an exercise program consisting of walking and swimming, activities that she enjoyed. As her conditioning improved, the amount of walking and swimming she could do increased.

Doris had questions about diet pills and whether they would be of value to her. While these may help in the beginning of a diet to curb the appetite, only good dietary habits and exercise can actually take off weight and maintain that weight loss. Also, diet pills do have medical risks that should be taken into consideration. Diet pills were not prescribed for Doris, and without them she did begin a slow but steady weight loss on her exercise and diet program. Such a gradual but nonetheless steady loss is far superior to a sudden crash diet. It is easier for the body to adjust to and is more likely to be maintained. When I last saw Doris she was exercising regularly, had lost fifteen pounds, and was wearing a size 12 dress.

ADEQUATE SLEEP

For the most part, older people maintain their energy and intellectual acuity best when they have seven to eight hours of sleep each night. Unfortunately, emotional problems such as grief, anxiety, or depression may interfere with their ability to get this much sleep. Emotional problems may cause the production in the body of agents called serotonins. These adrenalinelike compounds, which build up as the day goes on, frequently have the effect of waking a person after three to four hours of sleep. The body is tired, and the person goes to sleep, but when the body feels rested, the brain awakens the sleeper, due to the action of serotonins. What can help is to burn these off before bedtime by exercise. Thus, an evening walk, swim, or workout on an exer-cycle or rowing machine will not only help body tone and well-being but will also help you get a good night's sleep. On the other hand, if you do have a night in which you awaken, don't panic. Plan to take a short nap the next day.

ADEQUATE EXERCISE

An exercise program is helpful both in weight control and for ensuring adequate sleep, but there are many other benefits as well. Exercise helps tone the body, im-proves your energy level and sense of well-being, and helps relieves stress. If properly designed, it can help you maintain flexibility and balance. In addition, studies have shown that a good exercise program may help alleviate symptoms of chronic illness such as arthritis and cardiovascular disease. It also helps improve endurance, so that other activities may be enjoyed. Even the very elderly and partially disabled may ben-efit from daily short walks, swimming, dancing, or other forms of light exercise.

HORMONE REPLACEMENT THERAPY

While hormone replacement therapy is not for everyone, most women can derive many benefits to their health and well-being by using estrogen after menopause. (See chapter 6.) The major proven benefits at this point are the alleviation of symptoms of hot flashes and night sweats and the decreased risk of osteoporosis and arteriosclerotic heart disease. Other benefits include the strengthening of pelvic supports and improvement of bladder function, improvement of subcutaneous tissue (easing wrinkles), and the possible improvement of mental abilities and a decrease in the risk for Alzheimer's disease.

SUBSTANCE ABUSE CESSATION

Smoking

It is essential that any woman who smokes should take immediate steps to stop. There is no longer any question that smoking causes serious diseases and other health hazards and shortens life expectancy. It also decreases quality of life by causing respiratory diseases, high blood pressure, and stroke, not to mention the problems of cancer treatment and the threat that cancer itself causes to well-being. In addition, smoking ages the body more rapidly, causes wrinkles, and in general steals vitality.

Usually, for those who smoke fewer than ten cigarettes per day, the best way to stop is simply to stop. People who use these few cigarettes per day are probably not severely habituated, and with a modest amount of perseverance they can stop using cigarettes quite rapidly and without much difficulty. Those who smokes more than ten cigarettes per day should decrease the number of cigarettes they smoke in an organized program over weeks to months until they have gotten down to a daily intake of fewer than ten cigarettes. At this point they can stop, much the same as light smokers do. Decreasing the number of cigarettes can be done by carefully counting the number of cigarettes smoked and decreasing by one every two to three days. Many can be helped by using nicotine patches and nicotine gum. This should be done in consultation with a family physician, because these programs are somewhat expensive, and people should be given the best opportunity for success when undertaking them.

Alcohol

Several definitions exist for excessive alcohol use. Many of these depend upon other aspects of a person's life. A useful thing you can do to determine whether or not you have a potential drinking problem is to ask yourself if you are doing any of the following: drinking more than forty-five drinks per month, with a drink being defined as an ounce of whiskey, a glass of beer, or a glass of wine; binge drinking five or more drinks at a sitting; or repetitively becoming inebriated.

Alcohol use can be dangerous to the health in many ways. Its chronic use is the direct cause of illnesses such as liver disease, heart disease, and dementia. There are also the problems of acute use, such as traffic accidents that occur while someone is driving under the influence of alcohol, or falls or other accidents. Many social and relationship problems also may occur.

Drugs

Certainly the use of illegal drugs should be stopped, as only harm can come from such abuse. The guidance of a physician or other health care worker will probably be necessary to help overcome such habits. There are, however, other drug problems to be considered. These are the overuse or abuse of legal drugs, including prescription items and over-the-counter medications. Many people become dependent on such drugs and overuse them without realizing it. It is a good idea to take all medications that you are using, be they prescription or over-the-counter drugs, to your physician once a year for review. If you are overusing or abusing drugs, the physician can help you stop these practices. It is also important to be sure that the drugs you are using are not incompatible with each other. If such an incompatibility exists, you may have serious health risks you are not even aware of.

SAFETY

Some safety issues are obvious. For instance, you should always use a seat belt when riding in a motor vehicle. Most states have laws requiring this, and we have long understood the statistics proving that seat belts save people from death or serious injury. Other safety practices may not be as obvious. For instance, if you ride on a bicycle, motor scooter, motorcycle, or horse, you should wear a helmet. Accidents are more common as people age, and head injuries can be disastrous with respect to long-term health. There is little question that helmets reduce the number of head injuries that occur with these activities.

You should plan to to wear sturdy comfortable shoes to prevent stumbling and falling. In the 1940s and 1950s, four-inch heels were the style. Many women who are now in their sixties and seventies continue to wear these types of shoes. Most do not have the balance or the flexibility to continue this practice and should find lower heels that are still stylish for their everyday and dress use. It is also important to learn not to move too quickly, particularly on wet or waxed surfaces. As one ages, balance is not as good or as automatic as it has been, and decreased flexibility works against recovery from a slip to prevent a fall.

You should not undertake activities for which you no longer have the strength, stamina, reflexes, or flexibility. Thus, athletic activities you may have enjoyed at a younger age may not be in your scope at the present time. It is difficult to say in general what these may be, but the modification of your behavior to fit your abilities, although upsetting in certain situations, may be in your best interest in the long run.

Another safety consideration, often not even thought of, relates to the presence of firearms in the home. It has been estimated that 70 percent of American homes have firearms present. This leads to a large potential for accidental injuries.

In general, firearms should be kept unloaded and out of the reach of minors. If they are being used for protection and are to be kept loaded, their owners should be well schooled in gun safety procedures and should keep them away from all others who are not so knowledgeable. Certainly they should be kept out of the hands of violent and potentially violent individuals and those who are known abusers of drugs or alcohol.

Finally, avoid placing yourself at risk by modifying the defenses of your senses. For example, if you are out for a walk or a jog in areas where traffic is heavy, do not wear a Walkman, which will reduce your ability to hear potential dangers. Of course, if you note a decrease in your hearing or visual acuity, have these checked and proper therapy (glasses, hearing aid) implemented.

PREVENTIVE MEDICINE

Much of this book considers the importance of preventive medicine, what you should expect at your annual health maintenance visit, and how you can maintain good psychosocial health. While you may expect to receive a good deal of help from your health care professionals, seeking such help and adhering to the advice you are given is strictly your responsibility. Keeping you as young and healthy as possible for as long as possible is clearly a team activity, but you are the captain of the team.

CHAPTER 2

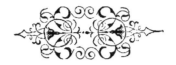

Your Annual Health Maintenance Visit

This chapter discusses the ideal components of the annual health maintenance visit. Your doctor may be limited by a busy schedule and may not be able to address each of these issues with you at each visit because of scheduling constraints, or because specific issues involving your immediate health needs may detract from considering all of them. Because of these possibilities, you may consider taking a little time before your visit to construct a list of items you wish to discuss with your doctor, much as you would prepare a shopping list before going to the supermarket. This ideal list should help you construct your own.

HEALTH HISTORY

Most physicians have you fill out a personal health history form, either before the visit or in the office at the time of the visit. This helps your doctor to make sure that all important information regarding your health is addressed. It also helps highlight specific areas of your health history that require special attention. It is a good way to be sure that all the bases are covered in an organized fashion. Some doctors now have you do this at a computer terminal in their waiting rooms. (See Table 2.1.)

The first portion usually relates to the chief complaint or the reason for seeing the doctor. In the case of a health maintenance visit, there may be no specific complaint, but if you have been noticing symptoms, this is a good place to begin. If you have a current complaint, the doctor will want to know when it began and under what circumstances it occurs. If you have developed a pain in some region of body, the characteristics of the pain and the circumstances under which it occurs, the things that make it worse, and the steps that you may have taken that give you relief will all be considered. You should describe in your own words your view of the complaint and then answer the specific questions that your physician asks relating to it. In this way your physician will get a better picture of what may be taking place.

TABLE 2.1.   Components of the Health History

Chief complaint

History of present problem

Past history

Review of systems

Gynecologic and pregnancy history

Psychosocial history

Occupation and avocations

Medications

Habits

Safety factors

Immunization history

The next area of your health history is your past medical history. You will be asked to list all of the serious illnesses and operations that you have experienced in the past. Such experiences may or may not have a direct impact on your current problem, but the information will help your physician to have a broader understanding of your overall health. You will also be asked how many pregnancies you have experienced, including term births, premature deliveries, miscarriages, terminations, and ectopic pregnancies. Pregnancy complications, types of deliveries, pregnancy outcomes with respect to the health of the baby, and other related information will be of interest to your physician and may also have an impact on your current health.

Your physician will take a gynecologic history, noting when you started menses, the frequency and length of your periods, when you went through menopause (if you have), and whether or not you are currently taking hormone replacement therapy. You will also be asked about related problems involving your menstrual history, such as abnormal vaginal bleeding, infections, surgical procedures required upon your genital tract, and a history of contraceptive medications or devices you may have used.

You will also be asked about control of urine and bowel movements and difficulties you may have that relate to either. Approximately 20 percent of women will suffer urinary incontinence during their lifetime, and the older the woman the more likely this is to occur. As many as 30 percent of residents in nursing homes complain of incontinence of urine. Likewise, bowel problems such as control of bowel movement and constipation are common problems that frequently plague older women. Many are embarrassed to discuss these aspects of their bodily function unless a physician questions them directly. Most of the time your physician will be able to offer methods to relieve these problems.

Physicians often ask general questions about your health as it relates to your organ systems in order to detect important information in a systematic fashion that may not have come out in the general discussion of your problems. This is called a review of systems.

Your physician will want to know about any medications that you have taken in the past or may be taking presently, which includes both prescription items and over-the-counter medications, the reasons for taking them, the doses, and any side effects or allergies you may have suffered.

Your physician will ask about the type of work you do and stresses you may be suffering in the workplace. A discussion of your hobbies and avocations may also shed some light on the symptoms you may be suffering or risks you may be taking with your health.

Your physician will ask about your use of alcohol and tobacco as well as other illegal drugs and should offer you some advice on curtailing such usage, discussing potential hazards to your health. Although you may feel you have heard all of this before, it is reasonable to listen closely, because the risks to your health from tobacco, alcohol, and illegal drug use are huge.

You may be asked questions regarding your living conditions—whom you live with and under what circumstances your household is constructed. There will be questions concerning your psychosocial well-being, potential stresses and emotional stress that you feel, as well as anxiety, depression, suicidal tendencies, and so on. Physicians now often inquire whether you have suffered physical or sexual abuse. Roughly 25 to 35 percent of women have suffered such problems in the past or are suffering them currently, and these types of emotional stresses can have a strong bearing on physical well-being.

You will be asked about your family and about the health of your parents, siblings, spouse, and children. Your physician will want to know about illnesses that may conceivably be familial or infectious diseases that may put you at risk because of close proximity to the ill person. If there is a familial tendency toward a specific condition, the physician may work with you to construct a family tree to get a better picture of the potential inheritance pattern you may be facing.

Your physician will probably discuss safety factors with you, reminding you to wear your seat belt and to use a helmet if you ride a bicycle, motorcycle, or horse, perhaps giving you some information on activities that may carry higher risks for you than they did when you were younger. Your physician may ask about the presence of firearms in the home and ask questions about safety precautions.

Finally, your physician will probably discuss your immunization records to be sure that you have proper immunizations for your age and risk circumstances. If you travel to foreign and exotic places, it is wise to make sure that you have the proper immunizations for those areas. Also, if you are planning a trip to a part of the world where there is malaria, you should ask about proper prophylaxis.

PHYSICAL EXAMINATION

Your general annual physical examination has eight components. (See Table 2.2.) It should begin with a blood pressure test. If your pressure is elevated, you should be

TABLE 2.2.	Components of a Physical Examination

Blood pressure

Height and weight

General physical

Breast

Pelvic

Rectal

Extremeties

Neurological

checked in the standing, lying, and sitting positions. If you are overweight or tall, a large blood pressure cuff will probably give a more accurate reading. The systolic blood pressure is the upper number of the blood pressure measurement, and the diastolic is the lower number. In general, systolic blood pressures below 140 and diastolic blood pressures below 90 are considered normal. Although blood pressure tends to rise slightly with age, your blood pressure levels from previous years should be considered. Generally, blood pressures are a bit higher when you are under stress, such as visiting the doctor. Repeat blood pressure tests at a later part of the examination may reveal a normal blood pressure.

Your weight should be checked and compared to that of previous years. If you are past the age of menopause, it is wise to have your height measured each year to be sure that you are not developing osteoporosis of your spine and thereby losing height. General evaluation of your hearing and of your vision should be carried out, and many doctors will look at your eye grounds with an ophthalmoscope in order to determine whether or not your retinal vessels are healthy. This is often a reflection of the vascular health of the rest of your body. Your general practitioner or your ophthalmologist should measure the intraocular pressure at least every two years to be sure that you are not developing glaucoma, and should inspect your pupils and their reaction to light. This will give some indication of your neurologic health with respect to these reflexes.

Your physician will probably palpate your neck to evaluate the size and consistency of your thyroid gland and look for any lymph nodes that may be enlarged. About 5 percent of women past fifty will develop thyroid disease of some sort, and the first indication may be an enlargement of one or both lobes of the gland.

Your physician will then listen to your heart and evaluate your heart rate (pulse). Although occasional irregularities of the heartbeat or skipped beats are normal, particularly as people get older or are under stress, gross irregularities of the heart rate may imply a conduction problem of the heart. Your physician may wish to investigate this and put you on therapy. Having a gross irregularity such as atrial fibrillation may lead to the formation of blood clots along the valves of the heart that may embolize.

This can have very serious health consequences if pieces of clots move to distant organs, such as the brain or lungs, and clog blood vessels in them.

Your physician will also listen to your chest to evaluate the sounds of your lungs as you inhale and exhale. Certain sounds in your lungs may suggest such chest conditions as pneumonia, bronchitis, or asthma.

Next, your physician will inspect and palpate your breasts, looking for irregularities, discolorations, and masses. Your physician should teach you to do breast self-examinations, and this should be done every month on a regular basis. If you find irregularities you should report them to the physician immediately. The breasts should be examined systematically, covering the entire breast as one would palpate the spokes of a wheel. By the end of the exam the entire breast and the subnipple area should have been palpated. Your physician may squeeze the breast to see if any material is excreted from the nipple, especially if you have experienced such secretions in the past.

Your physician will then examine your abdomen to be sure that there are no palpable masses or abnormalities in your internal organs. If scars are present on your abdomen and you have not discussed previous surgical procedures, you will probably be asked about their origin.

Your physician will then carry out a pelvic examination. It is up to you and your physician to decide whether or not to have a chaperone in the room, but your physician may automatically do this both for your comfort and to help with any procedures that may be necessary. You will generally be covered with a sheet, but this again is up to you and your physician. At all times your comfort and modesty should be taken into consideration. The physician will then observe your vulva to be sure there are no abnormalities of the skin or external structures. Any problems that you have noticed yourself should be brought to your physician's attention at this time. It is often possible because of pubic hair configuration for a physician to miss small lumps or lesions that you may be aware of. The vagina will then be examined with the use of a speculum. There are several sizes and shapes of speculums, and your physician will probably choose one depending upon your circumstances. In general, examination of virginal women is usually accomplished with a narrow Pedersen speculum, and some women with long vaginas will need a longer instrument to observe the cervix and the entirety of the vagina. At this point your physician will be looking at the mucosa of the vagina to detect any evidence of infection or other abnormalities. If an unusual or abnormal-looking discharge is present, the physician will probably take samples of the secretion for study under the microscope. It is possible in looking at these secretions to diagnose a yeast infection or an infection with a common vaginal organism such as trichamonas. It is also possible to observe the epithelium of the vagina under the microscope for evidence of bacterial infection.

The physician will then examine your cervix and probably, if it is an annual exam, do a Pap smear. Timed intervals for performing a Pap smear are quite variable depending upon your circumstances. If you are monogamous and have had three consecutive normal Pap smears, your physician may chose to repeat this exam only once every two years. If you have more than one sexual partner, or have other conditions that the physician may deem as high risk, an annual Papanicolaou test will probably be required. If your mother used diethylstilbestrol (DES) during her pregnancy and you were exposed in utero, you should have an annual Pap smear. If you have had a hysterectomy for noncancerous indications and your cervix has been removed, you probably require a Pap smear only every two to three years. Your physician may take cultures of your cervix if you are at high risk for a genital tract infection, but this is not necessarily done routinely.

Your physician will then remove the speculum and perform a bimanual exam, palpating your cervix, uterus, tubes, and ovaries in order to determine the size, shape, and consistency of your internal organs. In general, the ovaries of women past menopause shrink in size to approximately 2 cm (less than one inch in diameter) and retract toward the pelvic brim. Under these circumstances a physician will usually not be able to palpate the ovaries. If an ovary is palpable in a postmenopausal woman, the physician will probably order an ultrasound exam in order to decide whether or not it is enlarged and whether or not the enlargement is due to a cystic or a solid mass. Many women even past menopause will develop cystic ovaries, and, in most situations, they are benign. Nevertheless, the incidence of malignancy does increase with age, and such lesions in older women should be observed closely or investigated immediately.

The uterus also tends to decrease in size after the menopause. In premenopausal women, the corpus (body) of the uterus is usually two times the length of the cervix (2:1 ratio), but in older women the corpus size generally decreases, leading eventually to a reverse ratio of corpus to cervix (1:2). Also, if fibroid tumors have been present in the uterus before menopause, they will shrink in size so that the total premenopausal size of the uterus continually reduces after menopause. Uteruses that are growing in size after menopause must be further studied to rule out the development of a cancer.

Fallopian tubes are not normally palpable on pelvic exam either before or after menopause. If they are palpable they are almost always abnormal and should be further evaluated.

Your physician will then, more than likely, perform a rectal examination. Since colon and rectal cancers are quite common in older women, and a fairly large number can be detected by rectal examination, this is a worthwhile examination to have performed. During this exam, your physician will also be able to confirm findings from your vaginal examination and determine the strength of your rectal sphincter.

Your physician may perform an abbreviated neurological examination to determine whether or not your central nervous system is performing appropriately. The extent of this will probably be determined by your current history and any symptoms that you may be having. Your physician will also perform an exam on your extremities, noting such things as varicose veins, asymmetric muscle development, and skin abnormalities. Some evidence of the intactness of your circulation can also be obtained by palpating the pulses in the arteries of your lower extremities. Your physician will probably palpate your groin, looking for the possibility of enlarged lymph nodes and/or for evidence of hernias.

SCREENING LABORATORY TESTS

Screening tests are useful to detect diseases, particularly at their earlier stages. (See Table 2.3.) The Pap smear is excellent for detecting cervical cancer or precancerous

TABLE 2.3.   Important Screening Tests

Papanicolaou smear

Mammography

Hematocrit

Glucose (sugar)

Thyroid test (TSH)

Cholesterol (3–5 years)

lesions and may also detect cancers of other organs of the genital tract, such as the uterus and the vagina. It is not a good test for detecting cancer of the endometrium (uterus), as it will only detect about 50 percent of these. Nevertheless, if abnormal cells are found emanating from the endometrium, it is useful information for your physician to have.

Mammography is important for all women. The American Cancer Society guidelines indicate that a baseline should be performed sometime in your late thirties, and then mammograms should be performed every one to two years during the forties and every year after age fifty. If a woman has a strong family history of breast cancer, screening mammograms should probably be begun earlier and annual mammograms started at age forty. There is a good deal of controversy about how often mammograms should be performed. Some of this comes from the fact that young women or women on hormone replacement therapy have denser breast tissue than do other women and that therefore cancers may be missed. Nevertheless, if cancer is detected, the chances of its being detected at an earlier stage and successful treatment being possible is very strong. Therefore, all women should be offered mammography, depending upon their age and risk factors. Many women fear that the radiation they receive from mammography will actually increase their chance of breast cancer. This is very unlikely. Modern methods of performing mammography expose women to very little radiation. A recent study concluded that a woman who has annual mammograms beginning at age forty, has a ninetyfold benefit-over-risk advantage of the early detection of cancer (and survival) as compared with the risk that the radiation could cause a cancer.

An annual hematocrit is important to detect the possibility of developing anemias or other blood diseases. A fasting blood sugar done annually to detect evidence for diabetes mellitus is also useful since about 2 percent of the population will develop diabetes. Serum cholesterol should be performed every three to five years if your cholesterol is normal. An abnormally elevated cholesterol is frequently seen in women who have family histories of lipid or cholesterol problems, or who are suffering from diabetes, hypothyroidism, or some form of end-stage renal disease. As many as 5 percent of older women will develop thyroid disease, and an elevated cholesterol is often explained by performing a thyroid screening test, such as one for thyroid stimulating hormone (TSH). This test does not need to be done annually but should be done if the physician finds from your history or physical examination an indication that you may be hypothyroid, for instance, or if your cholesterol is elevated.

Women at risk for sexually transmitted diseases should be offered serologic tests for syphilis and other culturing that seems indicated by their history and physical findings. Women at risk for other medical conditions should be offered appropriate screening. Annual chest X rays and electrocardiograms do not seem to yield a very high rate of abnormal findings. Therefore, these tests are reserved for those who are at high risk for chest or heart disease.

IMMUNIZATIONS

Immunizations should be offered to each woman based on her risk factors. (See Table 2.4.) These immunizations should be offered to all older women:

1. Tetanus diphtheria booster—every ten years.
2. Influenza vaccine—annually beginning at age sixty to sixty-five.
3. Pneunomococcal vaccine—one dose at or about age 60–65, repeated every six to seven years.

Most people have been immunized against diphtheria and tetanus in childhood or young adulthood. If you have not been immunized, you should be. Once you have been immunized, a single booster shot every ten years will maintain your immunity to both tetanus (lockjaw) and diphtheria. Keeping your immunization up on these removes the risk of acquiring these conditions if you are exposed to them.

As a woman ages, her respiratory tract becomes more rigid, and it is more difficult for her to move mucus and overcome the effects of inflammation. Influenza is generally a three to four-day viral pneumonia; however, it irritates and inflames the bronchial tree and lung tissue to the extent that secondary bacterial infections often occur. These generally cause a higher mortality rate in older people. In any case, because the bronchial tree and lungs may be damaged to the point of causing breathing problems in the future, influenza vaccine given once a year can frequently help decrease your likelihood of getting influenza.

Likewise, pneumococcal vaccine which is a multivalent vaccine against Streptococcus pneumoniae, the organism that causes the majority of bacterial pneumonias, is worth getting. It is given after age sixty to sixty-five and should probably be repeated every six to seven years.

TABLE 2.4.   Immunizations for Low-Risk Individuals

Tetanus-diphtheria booster (every 10 years)

Influenza vaccine (annually)

Pneunomococcal vaccine (Every 6–7 years after age 60–65)

People at high risk for various conditions may need additional vaccinations. For instance, health care workers should be given hepatitis B vaccine because they may come in contact with patients with this serious condition. Those who have never been immunized against polio should be given a polio vaccine. Generally, older patients are given inactivated polio vaccine (IPV) rather than the oral type.

Finally, if you travel a great deal, you should be given specific vaccines against the diseases you may encounter in the countries that you visit. It is also important that you get antimalaria phrophylaxis if you are traveling to malaria-infested areas.

CHAPTER 3

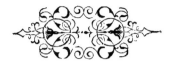

Nutrition: Eating for Good Health

The nutritional needs of an older woman are influenced by a variety of physiologic, psychological, and social factors. First of all, there is a general decrease in the need for calories, which begin gradually at about age thirty-five and mirrors the gradual change in ovarian function that begins in most women at about that age. Whereas an active young woman requires about 2,200 calories per day to maintain her weight, a woman over fifty requires about 1,700 to 1,900 calories per day. This will be modified one way or the other by the amount of exercise she gets and by the general state of her health. Chronic illnesses such as severe arthritis or respiratory problems will force a woman to limit her activities, thereby driving down the number of calories she needs. Medications may effect her metabolism or her ability to absorb nutrients. Such chronic conditions may force her into a vicious cycle whereby she becomes less active and therefore saves calories in the form of fat. With increased obesity her ability to exercise may further decrease.

Psychological factors may also be in play. As women age, the incidence of depression increases. Depressed individuals may overeat or spurn food. Also, with age comes loss, and with loss comes grief. Grief frequently is associated with loss of appetite. If a woman loses a spouse, her desire to prepare appropriate meals may fade and she may develop poor nutritional habits.

Social factors may play a role as well. A woman who is partially debilitated and living alone may have difficulty in obtaining the ingredients for nutritious meals. She may rely on foods high in starches, which are more easily stored in bulk, rather than obtaining fresh fruits, vegetables, and meats.

THE WEIGHT DILEMMA

The cold fact is that 35 percent of American women qualify as obese. This is in contrast to the fact that the ideal image of the American woman as depicted by such authorities as *Playboy* magazine and the fashion industry is that of a very thin woman. In order to maintain this image, fashion models are often drawn from the ranks of teenagers. Often clothing design has the thin woman in mind. This creates a difficult dilemma for most women, who try to stay thin and fulfill the image that is so popular. For many women this means strenuous dieting, with the risks of malnutrition. In younger women, anorexia nervosa and bulimia are common. Anorexia nervosa is seen when a woman's weight is 15 percent or more below the standard for her age and height. Bulimic women are not necessarily underweight, but they do use self-induced vomiting after eating, or cathartic purges. Thus, they are at risk for malnutrition. The risk for obesity is even greater as women age. Whereas women in their twenties have about a 20 percent incidence of obesity, for women in their fifties, the incidence jumps to 52 percent. Furthermore, there are cultural differences. Among adult women of all ages, the incidence of obesity is 47 percent for Mexican Americans, 48 percent for African Americans, and 32 percent for non-Hispanic whites.

There are many definitions of obesity. A reasonable one is that a woman is considered obese when she is 20 percent above her normal weight for her height. For many years, the standard was the Metropolitan Life Insurance Company chart. This standard was aimed primarily at those in the twenty-five-year-old age group, and it became apparent that it was inappropriate for older people. Figure 3.1 is a modified height/weight chart for women of all age groups. Note that the norms for older women are heavier than they are for younger women.

Mild obesity is defined as 20 to 40 percent above ideal weight. Generally, this poses little health hazard, and for most women it is merely a cosmetic problem. Weight loss from this degree of obesity is generally not difficult and can be managed by reducing the amount of fat in the diet and therefore the number of calories. Basi-

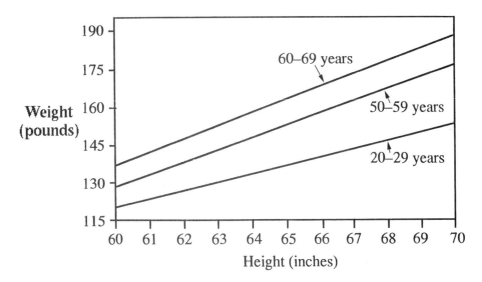

FIGURE 3.1.   Mean recommended weight for women.

cally, protein and carbohydrates yield 4 calories per gram, whereas fat yields 9 calories per gram. Thus, diets high in fat will be high in calories, and diets low in fat will be low in calories. Although it is recommended that people consume only 30 percent of their caloric intake in fat, the average U.S. diet has about a 34 percent fat content. Popular approaches, such as Weight Watchers and TOPS (Taking Off Pounds Sensibly), that reduce fat intake and portion size are reasonable ways for women with mild obesity to lose the pounds they would like to lose. As with anything else, developing good eating habits and maintaining a healthy weight is the challenge, one that most individuals cannot meet over the long haul.

Weights of 40 to 100 percent over ideal are considered moderate obesity. Clearly there is a great deal of leeway within this range, but the closer one gets to the upper end, the greater the risk of health hazards such as elevated cholesterol, heart disease, osteoporosis with fractures, and arthritis. Imagine what it would be like to be of normal weight and to be carrying a person of equal size around on your back all day. That is what 100 percent above ideal weight means. There will be a great deal of wear and tear on your heart, your joints, and so on. The good news is that individuals in the moderate obese category can lose weight with a good reducing diet and the emotional support of a health care worker, nutritionist, or diet specialist. The weight should be lost gradually, probably no more than four to five pounds per month, and the major concern is to develop new eating habits and adequate exercise so that the weight loss may be maintained. Appetite suppressants may be of value at least to get started; however, they may have ill effects for women with blood pressure and heart conditions and should only be used under the direction of a physician. They have been associated with pulmonary hypertension, a potentially lethal condition. They should not be used for long periods of time but only until the woman develops the eating and exercise habits that will allow her to continue her weight loss program. What must be avoided is rapid weight loss, followed by regaining, followed by rapid weight loss once again. These activities play havoc on the metabolism and often result in gall bladder disease and heart problems.

Individuals who are more than 100 percent above their ideal body weight are ranked in the severe obese category. Fortunately, they represent only about 5 percent of obese people. Their obesity is often associated with severe psychological problems, and generally they do not respond well to behavior modification. Frequently they require surgical procedures, such as stomach stapling, to reduce their capacity for food and their ability to absorb nutrients.

Some very thin women, who may be anorectic, generally suffer from a body image problem. They look in the mirror and see a fat person. Seeds of this were probably planted in their teens for a variety of reasons. Although the condition of anorexia nervosa can be physically very damaging and may even lead to death, many women have mild degrees of this and suffer into older age with the same body image distortion and the same restricted diet. During their menstrual years, they may have had an associated amenorrhea (absence of periods) or irregular menstrual periods and may have had difficulty achieving a pregnancy. This could very well have lead to a tendency toward osteoporosis because of decreased secretion of estrogen, and they may now pay the price in older age with fractures, particularly of the hips and wrists. In order to overcome this, behavior modification with respect to eating habits needs to take place. Problems of accomplishing this may be just as difficult for the underweight woman as for the overweight one.

A HEALTHY DIET

The U.S. Department of Agriculture and the U.S. Department of Health and Human Services have produced a joint publication, "Dietary Guidelines for Americans." It advises that you eat a variety of foods each day and balance the food you eat with physical activity aimed at maintaining and improving your weight (in the direction you may desire). It suggests that you eat plenty of grain products, fruits and vegetables, and a reduced amount of total fats, saturated fats, and cholesterol. It advises moderate use of sugar and salt, as well as moderation with respect to alcoholic beverages.

The guidelines recommend consuming foods from five major food groups every day. These groups and their daily recommendations are:

1. Vegetables (3–5 servings)
2. Fruits (2–4 servings)
3. Breads and cereals, rice, and pastas (6–11 servings)
4. Milk products (2–3 servings)
5. High protein food such as meats, poultry, fish, dried beans, peas, eggs, and nuts (2–3 servings)

Energy Status

The determination of a person's energy status takes into consideration dietary intake, usual weight, height, recent weight changes, and the influences of illness and medications. There are precise formulas for assessing ideal energy intake. These are generally based on weight, height, and age, with added consideration of activity level and disease states. With these formulas, a basal energy expenditure can be calculated and then calorie requirements determined on the basis of the individual level of activity. For instance, for someone with moderate activity, the caloric need would be 1.3 times the basal energy calculation. A person who is postoperative would require 1.1 times the basal requirement, but this would increase to 1.3 to 1.6 if there were an infection present, since higher degrees of caloric expenditure occur with fever and with the need to fight disease. For women over age fifty, the recommended daily allowance for calories is not age adjusted and is placed at roughly 1,700 to 1,900 calories per day.

Protein

In the United States, a high-protein diet has always been considered a healthy one. In fact, the average American adult consumes 1.5 times the recommended dietary allowance established by the Food and Nutrition Board of the National Research Council. There are many conflicting thoughts with respect to protein requirements for older Americans, but certain truths are agreed upon. For instance, protein stores diminish with aging, largely as a result of decline in lean body mass. Older people tend to lose muscle tissue unless they continue an exercise program. Total body protein production is also decreased in older people, but this depends on total body mass and therefore is quite variable. The level of serum albumin, the major protein in blood, declines with aging, so kidney function also gradually declines, affecting the way protein is broken down and excreted by the kidneys. There are those that feel that this decline in kidney function is not necessarily a normal component of aging but rather a damaging effect from long-term high-protein intake. As you may have guessed, there are differences of opinion on the significance of these various observations, but there is a fair amount of agreement that since decreased energy intake (total calories) may impair protein utilization, the elderly should consume only 12 to 14 percent of their calories as protein. The daily dietary allowance recommended by the Food and Nutrition Board of the National Research Council is 50 grams of protein for women past the age of fifty-one. Larger amounts are necessary for someone who is afflicted with certain illnesses or who is undernourished or has other circumstances that may be increasing protein loss.

Lipids (Fat and Cholesterol)

With aging, total body fat and serum cholesterol tend to increase. Part of this may be due to hormonal changes that influence fat and cholesterol metabolism, possibly because of a decreased turnover seen in advancing age.

The process of fatty deposits in the walls of arteries known as artherosclerotic accumulation begins in early life but seems to accelerate as people age. In women this is especially true after the ovaries stop functioning. Estrogen replacement after menopause appears to decrease the deposition of these plaques. There are probably several mechanisms by which this occurs. First of all, estrogen decreases total serum cholesterol and LDL cholesterol while increasing HDL cholesterol, the protective cholesterol. Second, estrogen seems to have an antioxidant effect on the plaques, helping to dissolve them. Third, there is good evidence that estrogen helps dilate coronary arteries. Plaque formation in coronary arteries can lead to heart attacks, so estrogen may offer some degree of protection in this respect.

Reducing dietary lipids and cholesterol is helpful in preventing obesity and its consequences in older women. Restricting fat and cholesterol in the diet of older people, however, has not been shown unequivocally to influence mortality rates from coronary artery disease, whereas estrogen use seems to be of value in this respect.

The recommendation for women over fifty-one years of age is that fat be limited to 30 percent of their total calories and that their cholesterol intake not exceed 300 mg per day.

Carbohydrates

The average diet of an older woman consists of 45 to 50 percent of calories from carbohydrates. Carbohydrates may be simple, such as simple sugars and complex. Because complex carbohydrates are often found in vegetables and grains, they also contain large amounts of vitamins and minerals and produce less stress on insulin release. Since Type II diabetes mellitus tends to increase with advancing age, having a higher percentage of complex carbohydrates in a diet may actually protect against this occurrence. It is recommended that older women consume 55 to 60 percent of their carbohydrate intake as complex carbohydrates.

Vitamins

Older people frequently suffer from vitamin deficiencies. The reasons for this are many. Often they decrease their food intake and do not eat a balanced diet that would ensure an adequate supply of vitamins of all types. In addition, they develop a thinning of their stomach lining, which may also cause a decrease in function, leading to atrophic gastritis. Associated with this is a decrease in acid production, changing digestive patterns and making absorption of nutrients more difficult. Older people often avoid sunlight, reducing the amount of vitamin D that their body produces. Other problems, such as the use of certain medications, the development of pernicious anemia, and increased alcohol use, all more common in the elderly than in younger people may lead to the inability to absorb or use vitamins and other nutrients. It is therefore fairly common for them to be deficient in all vitamins, but particularly vitamin B_{12}, folic acid, and vitamin D. On the other hand, fat-soluble vitamins such as vitamin A are rarely deficient in older people, because such vitamins are stored in fatty tissue and are quite high in conventional diets.

Vitamin B_{12} deficiency leading to pernicious anemia is seen in 5 to 10 percent of older people. Pernicious anemia is a condition that causes weakness, gait problems, diarrhea, and loss of appetite. To make the diagnosis, the physician measures the levels of vitamin B_{12} in the circulation. If some deficiency is found, the physician then looks further to try to find the cause of the deficiency. It is generally easily treated by supplementing the diet with vitamin B_{12} in pills or injections. Healthy adults should consume 2 mcg of vitamin B_{12} per day.

Serum folic acid levels are frequently found to be low in older people. This may occur because of poor dietary intake or poor absorption due to thinning of the gastric lining, but certain drugs and alcohol use may also interfere with folic acid absorption. Folic acid deficiency causes anemia, mental disorders disturbing normal thought processes, ulcers of the mouth, and diarrhea. Often, folic acid and vitamin B_{12} deficiencies coexist. The recommended daily dietary allowance of folic acid for healthy older adults is 200 mcg.

Vitamin D deficiency occurs because of lack of exposure to sunlight, poor dietary intake, and at times because of poor kidney function. It is quite common in older people. Vitamin D is involved with calcium metabolism and bone health, and deficiencies may speed the development of osteoporosis. The recommended daily dietary allowance of vitamin D for older people is 5 mcg. If the woman suffers from renal insufficiency, higher doses may be required as the vitamin D is lost in the urine when kidney function is poor.

Vitamins C and E and beta carotene may be of value because of their action as antioxidants. As such, their value in preventing coronary artery disease and certain types of cancer may be important. The actual proof of this is still not available. Supplementation is probably reasonable, and most multivitamin tablets contain appropriate amounts. The recommended daily dietary amount of vitamin E is 5 mg of alpha-tocopherol equivalents and 60 mg of vitamin C. The value of megadoses of these vitamins has yet to be proven, although large doses of vitamin E may help immune function in the elderly.

Niacin prescribed in large doses has been shown to reduce serum cholesterol in people with grossly elevated cholesterols. It should be given only under the supervision of a doctor and only to individuals who require it. The recommended daily dietary allowance of niacin for normal older people is 13 mg.

Although claims are made for beneficial effects from large doses of other vitamins and minerals, there is no scientific evidence of this. Certain vitamins in large doses can cause toxicity. Therefore, healthy individuals should limit their vitamin supplementation to the recommended daily dietary allowances. Table 3.1 summarizes these for vitamins and minerals. Table 3.2 lists foods that are good natural sources of vitamins and minerals.

TABLE 3.1.   Recommended Dietary Allowances for Women Over Fifty

Protein (grams)	50
Vitamin A (mg Retinol equivalent)	800
Vitamin D (mcg)	5
Vitamin E (mg alpha-tocopherol equivalent)	8
Vitamin K (mg)	65
Vitamin C (mg)	60
Thiamin (mg)	1
Riboflavin (mg)	1.2
Vitamin B_6 (mg)	1.6
Niacin (mg/niacin equivalent)	13
Folate (mg)	180
Vitamin B_{12} (mcg)	2
Calcium (mg)	800
Phosphorus (mg)	800
Magnesium (mg)	280
Iron (mg)	10
Zinc (mg)	12
Iodine (ugm)	150
Selenium (mg)	55

TABLE 3.2.   Some Food Sources of Vitamins and Minerals

Nutrient	Source
Vitamin	
A	Green, leafy vegetables, carrots, sweet potatoes, milk, liver
C	Oranges, lemons, grapefruit, strawberries, tomatoes, broccoli
D	Sunshine, fortified milk, fish liver oils
E	Green, leafy vegetables, wheat germ, whole grain cereals, vegetable oils
Folic acid	Oranges, strawberries, green, leafy vegetables, legumes, nuts, liver
Mineral	
Calcium	Milk, yogurt, cheese, sardines, salmon, kale, turnips, mustard
Iron	Meat, liver, dried beans and peas, iron-fortified cereals, prunes, prunce juice

Necessary Minerals

Calcium.   Osteoporosis is a frequent problem in aging. Estrogen replacement therapy can prevent or slow the process, but calcium supplementation either alone or in conjunction with estrogen therapy is also important. In order to have a positive calcium balance, women who are using estrogen replacement therapy need 1,000 to 1,500 mg per day of calcium. The average woman consumes 500 mg of calcium per day, so it is important that women plan for ways to improve this intake. The average quart of milk has 1,200 mg of calcium and equivalent other milk products are also a major source of calcium, but many women in their older years develop lactose intolerance and cannot use milk products or can only use them sparingly, but can use lactose-free dairy products. Therefore, calcium supplementation becomes very important. Calcium supplementation is extremely important for women who do not use hormone replacement therapy. It will not prevent osteoporosis in and of itself, but it may slow the process and in conjunction with weight-bearing exercise may offer relief to many women. Calcium supplementation can be obtained in a number of ways. Drugstores are filled with such preparations, ranging from inexpensive items such as Tums to quite expensive preparations. The important thing to remember is that you should consume 1,000 to 1,500 mg per day if you are on hormone replacement therapy and at least 1,500 mg per day if you are not. Adequate intake of vitamin D helps improve calcium metabolism. A recent study of healthy postmenopausal women demonstrated that supplementation with calcium and vitamin D reduced the risk of hip fracture by 43 percent and of other fractures by 32 percent. This was not as good as the result seen in studies with estrogen replacement therapy, but it was an improvement over the experience of older women not using estrogen.

Recently medications have been developed to help maintain bone integrity that are different from hormone replacement therapy. Calcium supplementation should be maintained with these drugs as well.

Iron.   A common cause of iron deficiency in older people is poor absorption of iron. Nevertheless, women who develop iron deficiency anemia should be evaluated for blood loss. Although they are no longer menstruating and no longer losing blood in that fashion, they may be losing blood from duodenal ulcers, colon cancers, diverticulosis, hemorrhoids, or from the gastrointestinal tract because of excessive use of aspirin or nonsteroidal anti-inflammatory drugs. In addition, elderly people tend to have diets that are low in iron. The recommended daily allowance of iron for an older person is 10 mg per day, which will allow for an absorption of about 1 mg daily. Certain things interfere with iron absorption. These include: excessive tea consumption, deficient amounts of vitamin C in the diet, and a decrease in stomach acid that occurs because of the atrophy of the stomach lining often seen in some older people. Anyone found to have an iron deficiency anemia should be evaluated for all of the conditions listed above before beginning iron supplementation therapy.

Zinc.   Zinc is a trace element but clearly a very important one. It has been implicated in such conditions as anorexia (poor appetite), abnormalities of taste, degeneration of the central area of the retina of the eye, poor wound healing, and dysfunction of T cells in the immune system. The recommended daily allowance of zinc is 12 mg, but elderly people rarely meet this requirement. To make matters worse, people with diabetes mellitus, those taking diuretics, and those using excessive amounts of alcohol are at greater risk for zinc deficiency. As with everything else, zinc absorption may be a problem for older people. Zinc has been demonstrated to be extremely important in the function of the immune system. It has also been shown to play a role in the healing of peripheral vascular ulcers on the extremities and to slowing the loss of vision seen in many of the elderly because of degeneration of the macular portion of the retina. It is important therefore to be sure that elderly individuals receive adequate zinc supplementation.

Chromium.   Although chromium has been shown to play a role in the increasing blood sugar seen in the elderly, and chromium deficiencies in rats have been associated with increased blood sugar, blood cholesterol, and opacities in the cornea of the eyes, its role in human aging remains controversial.

Selenium.   Selenium is probably an important trace element, and its deficiency has been linked to a number of diseases in older people, including cancer, coronary artery disease, and problems with immunity. Selenium concentration seems to decline with advancing age, and a high prevalence of cancer has been reported in areas where there is low concentration of selenium in crops. Animal studies have shown that diets high in selenium prevent cancer. Selenium and vitamin E have been shown to reduce radiation damage in cells that have been irradiated. The recommended daily dietary allowance for selenium is 50 to 200 mcg, but toxicity may occur in doses of 350 to 750 mcg. Toxicity is noted by a garlic odor on the breath, by nerve damage, and by changes in the fingernails. Therefore, while supplementing reasonable amounts of selenium may be prudent, the use of higher doses is not.

TABLE 3.3.   Drug Effects on Nutrients

Drug	Nutrient Loss
Aluminum hydroxide	Phosporus, calcium
Antacids	Thiamin
Anticoagulants	Vitamin K
Aspirin and nonsteroidal anti-inflammatories	Iron, fat, water-soluble vitamins
Cathartics	Calcium and potassium
Cholestyramine	Vitamins A,D,E,K, folic acid
Colchicine	Vitamin B_{12}, carotene, magnesium
Corticosteroids	Zinc, calcium, potassium
Digitalis	Protein, energy, zinc, magnesium
Furosemide (Lasix)	Calcium, potassium, sodium
Gentamicin	Potassium, sodium
Isoniazid	Pyridoxine
Levodopa	Protein
Methotrexate	Folic acid
Mineral oil	Fat, fat-soluble vitamins
Neomysin	Fat, protein, sodium, potassium, calcium, iron, vitamin B_{12}
Penicillamine	Zinc, Vitamin B_6, sodium
Phenobarbital	Vitamin D, folic acid
Phenytoin	Vitamin D, folic acid
Sulfa	Vitamin K
Tetracycline	Protein, iron
Trimethoprim	Folic acid

PLANS FOR GOOD NUTRITION

Older women should consume a diet of 1,700 to 1,900 calories per day, assuming that their weight is within the normal range. Obese women, particularly those whose weight is greater than 40 percent of ideal, should consider behavior modification with respect to diet, caloric intake decrease, and increase in exercise. Malnourished people (greater than 15 percent below ideal weight) should consider supplementing their diet to increase their weight closer to the ideal weight for their height. Alcohol abuse should be avoided, as it interferes with normal nutrition and absorption, and alcohol is frequently a calorie substitute for good nutritional intake. A supplementation of required vitamins and minerals is reasonable, but megadoses should be avoided. Adequate calcium intake should be maintained and vitamin D supplementation utilized. This is particularly important for those who are not using hormone replacement therapy but is important for all women. Anemias should be evaluated by a physician and appropriate therapy undertaken. Some medications may interfere with nutrition. Table 3.3 lists medications that are in common use and the nutrient loss that may be associated with them. Those who must take these medications may certainly wish to supplement these elements.

Good nutrition may be a problem in older people for a variety of reasons. A knowledge of the importance of good nutrition and the ingredients that go into it can help them plan an individual diet and dietary supplements, which can ensure good nutrition. This should be possible economically, using readily available foods and inexpensive supplements. Fad diets and megadoses of vitamins and minerals should be avoided. In many respects, you are what you eat, so it is worth your while to put some thought and energy into nutritional planning.

CHAPTER 4

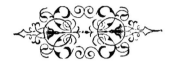

Exercise: Staying Fit, Flexible, and Limber

In youth, most women have endless energy and endurance, but with aging, many find that they have only enough energy to complete their daily activities and little of the physical reserve of energy that could be thought of as discretionary energy. In order to remain independent and to enjoy recreation and social activities, it is important for a woman to do everything she can to maintain an adequate level of discretionary energy.

As a woman ages, muscles throughout her body change. Her legs may become weaker. Her upper body strength may wane, and overall strength and endurance decrease. Chronic illnesses will also speed the decline of physical reserve. Pain that may go with a chronic illness such as arthritis will also contribute to declining activity and may speed the decline of physical reserve. Therefore, it is important for a woman to begin an exercise program early so that she may increase her energy reserve, decrease her tendency to fatigue, and thus get more enjoyment out of life overall. It is best to begin exercise training while a woman still maintains a high level of functional capacity. The earlier it is started the better, because investing energy in such a program pays energy dividends in the long run.

An exercise program is part of an overall approach to good health. It should be coupled with good nutrition and a healthy outlook toward life. Therefore, it should include an attempt to maintain time for fun and relaxation so that it may be a respite from the cares and other activities of the day. No matter how old a woman may be or how poor her general condition, an exercise program can probably be designed to increase her stamina and energy and strengthen her muscles. This is important; studies have shown that the most sedentary people have an increased risk of death from all causes at each age group than do people who are more fit. This means that low physical activity is an independent risk factor for increased mortality.

An exercise program has many benefits. It strengthens the musculoskeletal system and the heart and vascular system, improves muscle coordination, and helps the immune and endocrine systems. An added dividend is that it generally creates a feeling of mental and emotional well-being. Exercise may increase a sense of physical and physiologic well-being, and it has been shown, in many cases, to give symptomatic relief in many conditions by stopping or reversing the progression of a disease. At the very least it may improve function with no change in the disease.

The loss of muscle mass seen with aging can be reduced or reversed depending upon how intensely a person wishes to exercise. Also, exercise and diet control can alleviate the symptoms of adult onset diabetes and of obesity. It has been shown in those who suffer from rheumatoid arthritis and osteoarthritis that improved diet and exercise have caused improvements in pain-free function. Even in such disease states as chronic emphysema and obstructive pulmonary diseases, exercise programs have decreased the symptoms of shortness of breath and fatigue and have improved functional ability, even though pulmonary function tests were not improved.

There are different types of exercises, and choosing the proper one for individual needs or physical condition is important. Endurance training is weight-bearing exercise, which includes walking, jogging, stair climbing, cross-country skiing, and aerobic dancing; and non-weight-bearing exercise, which includes swimming, rowing, and upper- and lower-body cycle ergometrics. Resistance training may be of the low-intensity type, which is twelve to fifteen repetitions set at 40 to 60 percent of one maximum repetition, or the high-intensity type, which is eight to twelve repetitions at 70 to 85 percent of one maximum repetition.

Balance training includes static and dynamic exercises, including semitandem or tandem walking, balance beam, and posture training. Integrated exercises include several modes of training that require the use of both the mind and body in the performance of the exercises. Examples of this are hatha yoga, which integrates strength, flexibility, balance training, weight-bearing exercise, education, and relaxation; and tai chi, which integrates balance, weight-bearing exercise, and relaxation.

Whereas people can easily begin gentle programs of walking, dancing, aerobics, swimming, and so on, on their own and gradually increase their time and endurance, integrated exercise should be accompanied by proper coaching to ensure the greatest benefit with the least risk. Tables 4.1 to 4.3 list a number of conditions and the types of endurance and resistance training and integrated exercises that may be of help in alleviating symptoms.

ENDURANCE TRAINING

The heart is a muscle. With aging, its strength decreases, as does cardiovascular endurance. This is measured in terms of cardiac output, which is the heart rate per minute times the volume of blood that is pumped per beat plus the oxygen extraction at the muscle. Cardiovascular endurance decreases with age and is measured in the millimeters of oxygen per kilogram of body weight consumed in one minute. This is known as the VO_2 max. Between the ages of fifty and eighty, this may decrease between 25 and 35 ml per kg per minute. Also, maximum heart rate decreases with age on the average of one beat per year. Overall, there is a drop in maximum cardiac output that is age related. Sedentary activity has a greater effect on the stroke volume

TABLE 4.1. Recommended Endurance Exercise for Specific Medical Problems

Problem	Weight Bearing	Non-Weight Bearing	Coaching Recommended
Osteoporosis	+	—	—
Arthritis	+	+	+
Falls (tendency)	+	—	+
High blood pressure	—	+	—
Coronary artery disease	+	+	—
Peripheral vascular disease	—	+	+
Diabetes	+	+	—
Emphysema	+	+	+
Depression	+	+	—
Sleep disorders	+	+	+
Immune system dysfunction	+	+	—
Obesity	+	+	—
Incontinence	+	—	+
Muscle mass	+	—	—
Stamina	+	+	—

of the heart than on the ability of the tissue to extract oxygen. Thus, the VO$_2$ max decreases with age because of a decrease in heart rate, a decrease in stroke volume because of disuse, and a decrease in muscle mass. Fortunately, much of this can be reversed with an endurance muscle training program. Endurance training is the rhythmic contraction of large muscle groups at a specified heart rate for a specific duration of time. It may be weight bearing or non-weight bearing. Weight-bearing exercises have the added advantage of a positive effect on bone mass, particularly in the back and legs. Older people may not be able to participate in weight-bearing exercises because of musculoskeletal diseases involving the lower back, hip, knee, and ankle. These capabilities need to be taken into consideration when you design your own exercise program. If you suffer from a musculoskeletal condition that prevents you from performing weight-bearing exercises, perhaps you can consider non-weight-bearing exercises such as swimming or using a rowing machine or exercycle. Both non-weight-bearing and weight-bearing exercises will help improve your endurance. Studies show that regardless of age, cardiovascular endurance can be improved as much as 10 to 30 percent, depending upon the intensity of the training and the mode of training. The minimum recommendation for endurance training set by the American College of Sports Medicine is thirty minutes' accumulative exercise per day on at least three days each week. This is considered the minimum needed in order to raise an individual from the lowest sedentary level of the population, but it does not take into consideration the need for strength training, balance training, or any other form of activity. A reduction in fatigue is the principal benefit, and as you gradually feel better, you will be able to increase your endurance training to achieve greater benefits. You should consult your physician before beginning such a program to be sure that your heart and cardiovascular system can tolerate an increase in exercise. Even those who have had myocardial infarctions can benefit from endurance training, but this should be done under the direction of a physician.

RESISTANCE TRAINING

Muscles are comprised of two general types of fibers: slow twitch and fast twitch. Fast-twitch fibers are designed for rapid and powerful movements, usually those used in athletic activity. Slow-twitch muscle fibers are important for the usual body movements. Infants and young children have approximately 1.5 times as many fast-twitch fibers as slow-twitch fibers, but with age this ratio shifts, so that by age twenty the fibers are about equal in number. From then on, slow-twitch fibers exceed the number of fast-twitch fibers. Fast-twitch fibers are present in higher numbers if an adult woman maintains a high degree of athletic activity. Slow-twitch fibers remain constant because daily activities probably continue to strengthen them. Resistance training will improve both types of muscle fiber.

Often resistance training is ignored because of the time commitment necessary. To see an advantage, you should commit at least three months to this type of training. This will help you overcome the barriers of insufficient time and inconvenience and help you see the benefits of adding this to your daily routine. After three months of training, you can expect to see an improvement in your figure and strength, and an improvement in function in most of your activities. Resistance training for the most part involves weight lifting. There are a variety of programs, many of which are conducted by health clubs, that will help you through the initial steps. One program, Women on Weights (WOW), is available in many health clubs. For this program, the weight room is exclusively used by women, and trainers are available to assist in developing an individual program. Such weight programs are free with memberships in the clubs. An alternative to this would be to employ a certified personal trainer. This usually costs $25 to $35 per session, but many women team up with a partner and hire a personal trainer for the pair. The program should be set up to address the desired goals and past experience of each individual. Usually the training program consists of two training sessions per week for six to eight weeks, with follow-up sessions at various intervals.

With respect to resistance training, you will be able to increase the amount of weight you can lift and move through a full range of motion. As time goes on you will

TABLE 4.2. Recommended Resistance Training for Specific Medical Problems

Problem	Low Intensity	High Intensity	Muscle Specific	Coaching Recommended
Osteoporosis	—	+	Back muscles	+
Arthritis	+	—	—	—
Falls	—	+	Ankle	+
High blood pressure	+	—	—	—
Coronary artery disease	—	—	—	—
Peripheral vascular disease	—	—	—	—
Diabetes	—	—	—	—
Emphysema	+	—	Breathing muscles	+
Depression	+	+	—	±
Sleep disorders	—	—	—	—
Immune system dysfunction	—	—	—	—
Obesity	+	+	—	+
Incontinence	+	+	Pelvic muscles	+
Muscle mass	+	+	—	—
Stamina	+	—	—	—

realize an increase in strength and muscle mass. You will perceive a decreased effort for the same amount of work, and if you have been burdened by symptoms of depression, often resistance training helps alleviate them.

Resistance training, which is aimed at strengthening the pelvic muscles, may help those with incontinence problems. Exercises that improve diaphragmatic and chest wall musculature may help people with chronic lung disease. Improving strength in leg muscles may help balance problems and reduce the tendency to fall.

BALANCE TRAINING

Endurance training is primarily for the cardiovascular system, and strength training is primarily for the musculoskeletal system. Balance training primarily helps the neuro-

TABLE 4.3.   Recommended Integrated Exercises for Medical Problems

Problem	Balance Training	Range of Motion	Hatha Yoga	Tai Chi	Coaching Recommended
Osteoporosis	+	—	+	+	+
Arthritis	—	+	+	+	+
Falls	+	—	+	+	+
High blood pressure	—	—	+	+	+
Peripheral vascular disease	—	+	+	+	+
Emphysema	—	+	+	—	+
Depression	—	—	+	—	+
Sleep Disorders	—	+	+	—	+
Stamina	—	—	+	—	+

muscular system. It is closely interwoven with posture. Classically, many older women develop pathological posture, which includes flexion at the ankles, knees, hips, and elbows; a flattened lower back region; and an increased curvature of the thoracic spine. Other older women, however, have straight backs and good posture. This may have been helped by exercises such as sit ups, which improve abdominal muscle strength and therefore help alleviate low back strain, and by lifetime activities that have allowed these women to maintain flexibility and muscle strength. Balance training can be broken into static and dynamic components. Static exercises involve balancing the center of gravity while remaining in the same spot. This starts out with exercises that use a wide double-leg support and progressively narrows the base to a semitandem, to tandem, to single-leg support and to static two-leg support but rising onto the toes. It is also helped by sit-to-stand movements, rotation of the neck, or twists and side bending.

Dynamic balance is balance maintained during movement, and it can be made progressively more difficult by narrowing the base of support, side steps, crossover steps, forward and backward steps, high steps, heel-to-toe walking, and toe tapping. These exercises can frequently be accomplished as part of aerobic exercise classes or dance classes.

Range of motion of joints can be maintained or improved with gentle exercises that rotate each joint systematically at a relaxed pace. Range of motion can also be maintained during strengthening exercises in which the muscles used in the exercise surround joints. This may be done by performing dips or by incorporating these exercises into a dance program.

EXERCISE PROGRAMMING: WHERE DO YOU GET IT?

The amount of exercise you perform, the time you wish to give to your program, and your individual goals will all influence how much time you spend and what type of exercises you decide upon. Endurance exercises can be developed on your own and can be fitted to the things you enjoy doing. It is a good idea to have a checkup by your doctor before starting, so that you have some idea of the limits you may need to consider. The most desirable endurance exercises are those that are weight bearing, since they will help your skeleton to maintain its tone and perhaps cut down on the chances for developing osteoporosis. Resistance training will help improve your strength and stamina, and it will increase your muscle mass with the secondary advantage of improving your figure and general well-being. To get started, most women find joining the YWCA or a health club, or taking a few lessons with a personal trainer, to be useful.

Posture and balance training can be done on your own but probably, as a start, would be more enjoyable if you are part of a group. This too is available through YWCA or health clubs, or it could be more imaginatively obtained by joining a dance group. Community centers often have such opportunities available.

Most women prefer to develop an exercise program that integrates endurance, strength, and flexibility. This can be designed for time periods of from three days a week to daily. An example of a three-day-a-week plan would be thirty minutes of endurance, twenty minutes of strengthening, and twenty minutes of flexibility training each of three days per week. Combinations that fit your basic needs and availability of club or other activities could be, as an example, three days a week of endurance exercising thirty minutes, one day a week of a sixty-minute strength-building program (in a gym or other facility), and three days a week of flexibility training combined with or separate from endurance training. Whichever program you decide upon, remember these important guidelines:

1. Have a health checkup to be sure you exercise within the limits of your abilities.
2. Choose exercises that you will enjoy and are more likely to continue.
3. Set aside time in your busy schedule for exercise.
4. Seek professional or club help for strength and flexibility training.
5. If possible, get a buddy to work with you. This will make your exercising more fun and will help ensure that you continue.

CHAPTER 5

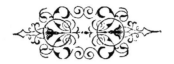

Things to Know About Medications

We are fortunate to be living in an era when many diseases and unpleasant symptoms can be treated with available medications. Also, technology has advanced to the point where researchers can often devise medications for specific needs. Thus, it is a rare person who is not exposed to a medication in some form at frequent intervals.

Older people may have difficulty with medication use for several reasons. First of all, older people tend to have more diseases and conditions than do younger ones. This generally means that they will have more medications prescribed for them and also may be more likely to use over-the-counter medications. With an increasing number of exposures, the opportunity for adverse reaction or drug-to-drug interreactions is greater. One study showed that 15 percent of an elderly population took two or more prescription medications daily. Another reported that 87 percent of those over the age of seventy-five were receiving drug therapy regularly, and 34 percent were using three or four drugs daily.

Second, older people may have an increased vulnerability to medications because of the effects of the aging process. Because of a change in their cell and organ metabolism, they may use and detoxify medications at a slower rate than do younger people. Also, because of impairments of liver or kidney function, they may detoxify and excrete drugs more slowly.

Finally, because of the aging process, older people may not utilize their medications properly. Because of hearing impairment, they may not understand the explanations given to them by doctors, pharmacists, or other health care workers for the appropriate use of their medication. With visual impairment, they may have difficulty reading instructions on the label, and with memory impairment, they may either forget instructions or even forget whether or not they took the medication. All of these problems make them more vulnerable to adverse drug reactions.

To understand why medications may affect an older person differently than they do a younger one, one must consider the changes in physiology that may contribute to this problem. First of all, there may be problems in absorption of a medication. Several reasons are possible for this, including a change in the acidity of stomach fluid; a change in the emptying time of the stomach, which is usually more sluggish in an older person; the decrease in intestinal motility that is frequently seen in older people; a change in the secretion of gastrointestinal fluids both in volume and composition; impairment of blood flow to the intestines, which is necessary to carry off the medication once it is absorbed; the possible presence of gastrointestinal disease, and overall individual general health.

Although the acidity of stomach juices decreases to a greater degree in women than in men as they age, the actual importance of this is difficult to understand. It is possible that some pills and capsules will dissolve more slowly because of reduced acidity, and under certain circumstances a physician may wish to prescribe a medication in a liquid rather than pill form if it is known that the patient has a decrease in acidity. Of greater risk, however, is the fact that with multiple drug use, multiple drug interreactions may reduce absorption.

The second condition that can influence drug usability in older people as compared to younger ones has to do with the change in body tissue content. Total body water and blood volume tend to decrease with aging. Since muscle mass tends to decrease, there is a relative increase in body fat; body fat increases from 33 to 45 percent in older women. Fat-soluble drugs are more readily stored in older patients, meaning that less of the drug is available for use in a single dose and that the active time the drug will function is increased, because it will be slowly removed from the fat storage areas. Liver size also decreases with age, thus, medications that are detoxified by the liver will have a longer life in the body in older people than they will in younger people. Different drugs are metabolized at different rates. Studies of several drugs detoxified by the liver have shown an increased half-life in the body of from 29 to 78 percent in older individuals. Half life is the time it takes for one half of the dose of the drug to disappear or be detoxified.

Kidney function also decreases with age. Therefore, drugs that are eliminated by the kidneys will stay in the body for longer periods of time and will continue to be active.

On the other hand, some medications act completely differently in older individuals than in younger ones. An example are those that affect the body's beta-receptors, which are found in several areas of the body and help to regulate many body functions, including blood pressure and heart rate. Medications that work on beta-receptors, such as certain blood pressure medications including propanolol, have a decreased activity in older people, probably because of a decreased affinity of beta-receptors to attach these drugs.

Most older people require lower doses of medications for the usual response and often will have toxic reactions at doses typically used in younger individuals. An example of this is the use of the sedative agent diazepam (Valium) in patients being prepared for dental or other procedures. It was noted that patients aged eighty or over required an average dose of 10 mg compared to 30 mg for patients aged twenty. Another example is warfarin, a blood-thinning medication used for anticoagulation.

Older people may be more or less sensitive to drugs. In general, opiates, sedatives, barbiturates, and anticoagulants will usually be required in lower doses than before, whereas certain of the beta-blockers may be required in higher doses. It is therefore important that your doctor take these factors into consideration and individualize the medications and doses that are prescribed for you.

ADVERSE EFFECTS OF MEDICATIONS

It is difficult to define whether or not a medication is having an adverse effect on a given individual. Healthy human beings have multiple irritating complaints and discomforts during a typical day. For instance, under certain circumstances, someone may suffer a variety of aches and pains, fatigue, inability to concentrate, inability to fall asleep, irritability, and mild depression. In fact, a large study on a college campus that compared complaints kept in diary form by a group of students taking no medications with a group who were on various medications actually found that the symptoms they complained about were similar. Nevertheless, adverse drug reactions are reported more frequently and in greater severity in older patients. For instance, one study showed that about 10 percent of patients in their twenties will suffer adverse drug reactions, whereas 25 percent of patients over the age of eighty will have such experiences. A study on nonsteroidal anti-inflammatory drugs looking at the effects on gastrointestinal bleeding and suppression of the blood-producing system found that 75 percent of all reported adverse reactions, and 91 percent of all fatal complications, occurred in those over the age of sixty.

It is important for anyone who is about to take a prescription medication or an over-the-counter remedy to consider the following: What is the natural history of the problem? Is there an actual hazard to life or health if the condition is left untreated? A good example of this is a viral illness such as the common cold. While it can frequently make a person feel quite ill, it is generally self-limited with respect to time, and in most cases there are no medications that will alter its course. The best that one can hope for is to get symptom relief, so medications that give symptom relief should only be used if they are not likely to cause an adverse reaction. Everyone has a runny nose and sneezes a great deal with a cold. Vasoconstricting agents such as Afrin, Neosynephrine, and ephedrine give relief for these symptoms; however, they frequently cause increase in blood pressure, and this may be quite dangerous for older people with compromised vascular systems, particularly those who already know they have hypertension. Thus it may be better to put up with the stuffy nose than to run the risk of an adverse vascular accident. Likewise, using antibiotics to treat a viral infection is probably a waste of time, because viruses are not susceptible to antibiotics. A potential adverse reaction to antibiotics might be the development of a superinfection, because protective bacteria are killed off. Another adverse reaction might be the development of an allergy to the antibiotic that would preclude its use in the future when it might actually be needed.

The second thing to consider is whether or not the medication will be effective against the disease the person has at the time the medication is taken. As an example, relatively mild nonsteroidal anti-inflammatory drugs such as aspirin, ibuprofen, or naprosyn may be useful in mild cases of arthritis in the usual over-the-counter doses. For an advanced arthritis, more potent therapy such as corticosteroids or higher doses of more potent nonsteroidals may be necessary. A person who tries to self-treat an advanced form of arthritis with an over-the-counter nonsteroidal anti-inflammatory drug may be exposing herself to the risks of the drug, such as gastrointestinal bleeding, without receiving any of the benefits. Likewise, if the usual dose does not work, some people might tend to try a higher dose, which would increase the chances of an adverse reaction and might not necessarily provide the pain relief desired.

Finally, some people are hypersensitive to medications even at the usual prescribed dosage. Thus, what normally would be an appropriate drug at an appropriate dose for the average individual might actually cause a hazard for someone with a hypersensitivity. All humans are different, and their responses to medications have the potential of being variable.

Many medications will have a positive effect on a disease condition but may exert an unfavorable effect on the quality of life. Some of the side effects of common medications used in treating problems of the elderly are specifically due to the action of the drug and may limit the ability of the individual to function in normal society. These side effects may be a decrease of initiative, impaired memory, disturbed sleep patterns, increased fatigue, and impaired sexual function. Many drugs can cause psychiatric symptoms, including confusion, disorientation, hyperactivity, hallucinations, and depression. Cimetidine, a compound found in many medications used for gastrointestinal upset, often causes mental confusion in the elderly. Sulfa drugs have been known to cause psychosis and delirium. Tranquilizers and antihypertensive drugs have caused memory and thinking impairments in some elderly individuals and have actually caused symptoms that are similar to those seen in Alzheimer's disease. Antihypertensive drugs often cause sexual dysfunction, and this has been seen with a wide variety of such drugs including thiazide diuretics, as well as drugs that work on the central nervous system and those that block the beta-receptors. Tranquilizers and antidepressant drugs have a similar potential, and some may affect the pituitary gland in such a way as to cause breast secretion. This is often associated with decreased libido and may cause impotence in men. Many drugs found in antispasmodic, anti-Parkinsonian, antihistamine, muscle relaxant, and antiarrhythmia medications may also cause sexual dysfunction, usually a loss of libido. While these drugs may affect younger individuals in a similar way, the likelihood of such adverse reaction is more common in the elderly.

ADVERSE REACTIONS CAUSED BY DRUG-DRUG INTERREACTIONS

Drug-drug interreactions are more common in older people because of the change in their physiology and the fact that they tend to take more medications than do younger people. There are many reasons that these interactions may take place. For instance, a drug may change the rate of absorption and hence the bioavailability of another drug; a drug may increase or decrease the rate of metabolism; a drug may decrease the rate of excretion of another drug; or a drug may influence the way another drug bonds to tissue in the body, thereby changing the bioavailability of that drug in the circulation. For example, a person taking iron may not absorb an antibiotic of the tetracycline family adequately because the iron binds these medications in the stomach. The GI medication cholestyramine may reduce the absorption of such important agents as thyroxin, Coumadin, or thiazide diuretics. If a drug requires stomach acidity to be absorbed, someone using an antacid may not absorb a prescribed dose properly.

Changes in GI motility may influence the absorption of the drug from the intestinal tract. Drugs that delay stomach emptying may prevent the absorption of another drug from taking place. An example of this is one of the atropinelike compounds, Pro-Banthine. Since this slows stomach emptying, it prevents pain medications such as acetaminophen from being absorbed. On the other hand, medications that increase the speed of stomach emptying may actually allow such agents to be absorbed more rapidly.

Another interesting drug association often seen in the elderly is the relationship of a digitalis compound, digoxin, with bacterial activity in the colon. Bacteria in the colon deactivates digoxin in about 10 percent of patients. Thus, when antibiotics that destroy colon bacteria are given to them, digoxin plasma levels rise, which may have a toxic effect.

Many drugs induce enzyme activity in the cells of the body. Examples of these are phenobarbital, glutethimide, and some of the anticonvulsant drugs. This may speed up the metabolism of other medications and thereby shorten the period of time that they would be active. One dangerous adverse association is found when someone takes one of these agents plus Coumadin. The active period of Coumadin will be shortened because of the increased enzymatic activity caused by these medications, and its anticoagulation effect may be compromised. This could lead to a clotting problem.

Some drugs decrease the ability of the kidneys to eliminate another drug. This is more common in older people whose kidney function may be decreased. Other drugs may actually speed the loss of another drug from the circulation because of increased renal activity.

HOW TO DECREASE THE CHANCE OF ADVERSE DRUG REACTIONS

1. Bring all of the drugs you are taking, both prescription and over-the-counter, to your physician for evaluation. Remember to tell your physician about your use of tobacco, alcohol, caffeine, laxatives, and pain and sleep preparations. It is often easy to forget something that you have been taking for years when you discuss medications with your physician.

2. Take only medications that you clearly need. Discuss with your doctor why a medication is being prescribed and what may be accomplished by your taking it. Doctors are human beings. If you go to them with a complaint, their tendency is to do something to alleviate this complaint. What the doctor may not know is how serious a problem this may be to you. Take a few minutes to discuss this more fully with your doctor so that you are not given medications you could get along without.

3. Be on the lookout for any unusual new symptoms that you did not have prior to taking the medication. Check with your doctor if you do notice any unusual symptoms to be sure you are not developing an adverse reaction. If you are unable to reach your doctor and are not sure about your symptoms, it is probably best to stop the drug unless it has been prescribed for a life-threatening illness. After consulting your doctor, you can always restart it.

4. You should always take the lowest dose possible initially and should not increase the dose beyond what is prescribed.

5. If you are not sure about the instructions for the medication, ask your doctor to give you written instructions and be sure that the pharmacist clearly labels the medication with its name and dosage schedule. Be sure that the pharmacist is aware of other medications you may be taking so that you can be advised about a potential drug-drug interreaction. Before leaving the pharmacy, be sure that you can read the label and that you understand what you are to do. Also, make sure the pharmacist has placed the medication in a container you can open.

6. If you are being given a medication that requires multiple dosing per day, work out a system to remember that you have taken the medication. There are special boxes that you can purchase at the pharmacy for putting out your daily doses of a medication. It is easy to forget whether or not you have taken the medication and therefore either to double dose or to miss a dose. Also, try to fit the drug-taking schedule into your daily personal schedule. It is often easier to remember to take a medication at mealtimes than to take one at an odd hour in the middle of the morning or the afternoon if the drug can be safely taken with food.

7. If you are taking a drug that requires careful monitoring, such as the anticoagulation agent Coumadin, or the antidepressant lithium, be sure to keep the scheduled appointments to have your plasma levels tested. Many of these agents have a very narrow margin between therapeutic levels and toxicity.

8. Finally, if you are using homeopathic medications that you purchased from a health food store or some other source, be sure to let your physician know what you are taking. Many of these are quite potent and can cause an interreaction with other medications you may be taking. Also, they may have a pharmacologic effect that is contraindicated for you. The fact that something is considered "natural" does not always mean, in your case, that it will be safe. Be careful with such remedies.

It is not my aim to frighten you or prevent you from using medications that you need; quite the contrary—to maintain good health it is often necessary to use pharmacologic agents. It is important to understand some of the potential hazards that the use of pharmacologic agents can cause. You have important resources in your physician and your pharmacist; be sure to use them. Remember that it is prudent to use only the medications you need and to use them properly and as prescribed.

CHAPTER 6

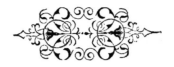

Things to Know About the Menopause and Hormone Replacement Therapy

Menopause is defined as the time when menstrual periods cease, but there is a peri-menopausal period, which probably starts at about age thirty-five. From this point on, the ovaries begin to fail, although the change is usually gradual. It is not uncommon for menstrual cycles to change in length and for periods to change in number of days and type of flow at some time after the age of thirty-five. It is also quite common for women to note poor reproduction efficiency after thirty-five. They may have more difficulty in getting pregnant and a higher percentage of miscarriage. The ovaries are changing, and their function is not as efficient as it was in the earlier years.

Not every menstrual cycle in this period of life is associated with a successful ovulation, and the amount of estrogen and progesterone produced during the cycle may be variable. This may lead to improper maturation of the lining of the uterus (endometrium), and women may experience some abnormal uterine bleeding in the form of heavier or lighter periods, longer or shorter periods, or bleeding between periods. Also during this time, 30 to 40 percent of women may develop benign smooth muscle tumors called fibroids (leiomyomas). These tumors grow in concentric circles as onions do, laying down layer after layer of cells. This kind of tumor does not have a direct blood supply, so as it grows larger, the center of the tumor may die. Over time it may actually calcify. When degeneration occurs, women often suffer lower abdominal pain. Also, the fibroids may press upon the lining of the uterus, interfering with normal endometrial function. This may give rise to abnormal uterine bleeding. If a fibroid happens to be located just beneath the lining of the endometrium (submucous myoma), it is more likely that abnormal uterine bleeding will take place. The menstrual period is often associated with abnormally heavy uterine bleeding, perhaps pain, and in some cases, an enlargement of the uterus.

Most uterine (endometrial) cancers develop in the lining of the uterus and occur after menopause. Perhaps 5 percent occur in the last ten to fifteen years of menstrual function. Women over thirty-five who have abnormal uterine bleeding are generally evaluated with an endometrial biopsy to be sure that no malignancy is present. Physical examination and ultrasound examination will allow the doctor to determine whether or the not the uterus is enlarged, whether there is an irregularity affecting the endometrial lining, and whether such conditions as polyps or fibroids are present. If these are found, the physician can determine the therapy that will alleviate the symptoms. It is important to rule out disease before attempting to treat abnormal bleeding of the perimenopausal period.

If the biopsy shows benign tissue, and the evaluation of the patient shows no fibroids or other abnormalities, it is reasonable to regulate the menstrual cycles during the perimenopausal years using hormone therapy. There are several different ways of doing this, and no one way is best for every patient. For a woman who is not ovulating regularly, it is possible to prescribe a progesterone compound for the last ten days of her menstrual cycle. This allows a ripening of the lining of the uterus and a more reasonable menstrual flow after the hormone is withdrawn. For the majority of women this will suffice. For those women for whom this does not work, and for those with irregular menstrual periods during this time, the use of birth control pills may be the answer. Most birth control pills are synthetic estrogen and progesterone hormones that may be given in a constant dose of both estrogen and progesterone each day throughout the month (monophasic pills) or in varying doses of estrogen followed by estrogen and progesterone in order to mimic a normal menstrual cycle (biphasic or triphasic pills). It probably does not matter which pill is selected during this time. Most physicians will select a relatively low-dose monophasic pill, which ensures a relatively thin endometrial lining and therefore minimum bleeding during menses. The use of such pills prevents large fluctuations of hormone produced by the ovaries and, therefore, fluctuations in the thickness of the endometrial lining that may lead to heavier bleeding.

Oral contraceptives are much more potent than are the hormones used in hormone replacement regimens after menopause. The estrogens and progesterones are usually synthetic and are four or more times more potent than the natural estrogens that are generally used in the postmenopausal period. They should not be given to women who are smokers. An epidemiologic relationship between the use of oral contraceptives in smokers after the age of thirty-five with heart attack (myocardial infarction) has been noted. Such a relationship is not seen in women over thirty-five using oral contraceptives who do not smoke. The problem may well be simply that smoking causes an increase in myocardial infarction in this age group, but, for now, it is best to avoid oral contraceptives in smokers of that age.

The use of oral contraceptives to regulate menstrual flow in women over thirty-five is actually very reasonable. First of all, in the absence of pathology, they do the job. Second, there are many other health benefits to be enjoyed by the user. The incidence of both endometrial and ovarian cancer is reduced greatly in oral contraceptive users, and this benefit continues throughout life. There are the obvious advantages of decreased menstrual flow and therefore decreased blood loss, and there may be an advantage for improved bone mineralization in oral contraceptive users. The FDA has approved the use of oral contraceptives until menopause in healthy women. For the nonsmoker, this is probably one of the better ways to proceed.

A third way to alleviate the symptoms of irregular menses in women over age thirty-five who have no obvious pathology is the use of continuous progesterone. Progesterone can be given to smokers, because it is apparently the effect of estrogen that may be related to association of smoking, oral contraceptives, and heart disease. Progesterone may be given in two different ways: as a continuous daily oral dose such as seen in progesterone-only oral contraceptives or by injection with Depo Provera. After four to six weeks, the Depo Provera will generally cause the patient to have no further menstrual periods. It is injected about every three months. The oral preparation may lead to mild periods that may be irregular or to a cessation of periods altogether. The decision about which preparation to use should be made by you and your doctor, taking into consideration your particular needs and the potential side effects you may have experienced from these preparations in the past. If you are taking the oral contraceptives as a means of controlling abnormal uterine bleeding in the perimenopausal period, your physician can test your pituitary hormones, FSH and LH, during the week you are not taking the pills. When these pituitary hormone levels become elevated, you have probably gone through menopause and can be switched to hormone replacement therapy if this is what you and your physician desire. It is not reasonable to start hormone replacement therapy before menopause. Unlike the oral contraceptives that modulate ovarian function by preventing ovulation and thereby control the development of the lining of the uterus, the estrogen and progesterone used in hormone replacement therapy do are not interfere with ovulation, are additive to hormone production by the ovaries, and are not contraceptive. Women who begin replacement therapy during the perimenopausal period actually may have heavier periods and more irregular bleeding than before, and can even conceive.

MENOPAUSE

Menopause is defined as the cessation of menstrual periods. It occurs in the average woman at about the age of fifty-one. There is certainly a spectrum, and premature menopause can occur even in the twenties, whereas some women will continue their menses until close to age sixty. Considering the increase in longevity modern women enjoy, about one third of the average woman's life is lived after menopause.

Often menses do not cease abruptly. Women may experience irregular menses with skipped periods over several months. Therefore, most physicians do not consider that menopause has occurred until at least six months have passed without periods. The pituitary hormones, follicle stimulating hormone (FSH), and luteinizing hormone (LH) rise rapidly during the first twelve months of menopause and then level off. A return to ovarian function, as may happen when an occasional period occurs after menopause, may be enough to reduce these hormones for a short time. But the mere fact that FSH and LH are elevated is not definite proof that the woman has completed menopause. Hormone replacement therapy at the doses that are usually given, however, will not appreciably influence FSH or LH levels.

Major changes in a woman's body may occur in the period of time after menopause. As can be seen in Figure 6.1, when age is considered a continuum, the first symptoms that occur generally at the time of menopause are hot flashes and night sweats, usually accompanied by dryness of the vagina. No one is quite sure why women have hot flashes or night sweats. Several important body functions are regulated in the brain, in

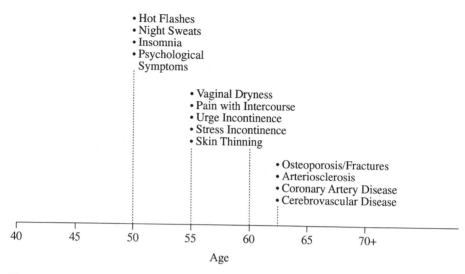

- Hot Flashes
- Night Sweats
- Insomnia
- Psychological Symptoms

- Vaginal Dryness
- Pain with Intercourse
- Urge Incontinence
- Stress Incontinence
- Skin Thinning

- Osteoporosis/Fractures
- Arteriosclerosis
- Coronary Artery Disease
- Cerebrovascular Disease

```
40        45        50        55        60        65        70+
```

Age

FIGURE 6.1.

the area called the hypothalamus. It controls the pituitary function, which regulates ovarian function. Small polypeptide substances, the gonadotropin-releasing hormones (GnRH), are produced in the hypothalamus and are responsible for the production of FSH and LH, which are important for the regulation of ovarian function while a woman is in her menstrual years. Because the ovaries produce no estrogen after menopause, there is no feedback to modulate the FSH and LH, and their levels rise. This undoubtedly has an effect on the hypothalamus as well. The temperature control centers of the body also have a regulatory area in the hypothalamus, perhaps adjacent to the gonadotropin-controlling area. This may be why menopause has an effect on the temperature-controlling mechanism. Because the body receives the false information that the body temperature has risen, it stimulates the dilation of blood vessels in the skin to release heat. Perspiration is usually part of this mechanism. The body temperature may then drop as much as a whole degree. At this point, the temperature control center realizes that the body temperature has gone too low and stimulates muscle activity to create heat and thereby raise the temperature back to normal. A typical hot flash consists of a dilation or flushing of the skin, increased perspiration (or night sweats), followed by a chill, which is actually an increased muscle activity. Stress and nervousness may aggravate this function. Not all women experience hot flashes and night sweats, but enough do to make it a common problem. Estrogen replacement therapy quickly alleviates this unpleasant symptom.

Vaginal dryness is due to the fact that there is less vaginal secretion after menopause, and this too can be alleviated by either oral or vaginal estrogen therapy.

Hot flashes and night sweats often awaken women who have them, leading to sleeplessness, fatigue, and nervousness. The problem of vaginal dryness may lead to discomfort during intercourse and then to a loss of libido. It is difficult to relate any of these symptoms statistically to menopause. They are probably secondary symptoms in certain women, depending upon the degree of discomfort that the primary symptoms cause. About 75 percent of American women report hot flashes and night sweats, and about 15 percent of these women report that these are severe. Only about one fourth of these women will continue to have such symptoms for as much as five years, and about fifteen percent will continue to have them through most of their lives. Somewhere between 20 and 38 percent will complain of vaginal dryness and the discomfort with intercourse that is associated with it.

Both the vagina as well as the urethra and bladder neck are sensitive to estrogen, and their tissues become atrophic when estrogen is withdrawn. This may lead to a decrease in the ability of the urethra to hold back the flow of urine because of a 30 percent reduction in the urethral closure pressure, and it may lead to symptoms of urgency and frequency of urination. Furthermore, the supporting tissue of the pelvic organs is dependent on a material called collagen, and the production of this is stimulated by estrogen. Therefore, over time, the bladder, bladder neck, urethra, and pelvic organs may lose their support and prolapse into or out of the vagina leading to a cystocele, rectocele, or the prolapse of the uterus itself. Estrogen is important in maintaining pelvic support.

Also, because of a loss of collagen from the subcutaneous tissue of skin, after menopause skin thickness decreases at about 1.2 percent per year, and the amount of collagen within the skin is reduced about 2.1 percent per year after menopause. This can be partially reversed by estrogen therapy. Comparison studies that have been done of postmenopausal women who have been on estrogen or placebo control have demonstrated a significant difference in thickness of the skin and subcutaneous tissue, favoring those on estrogen therapy. Clearly the more rapidly subcutaneous collagen is lost, the more rapidly wrinkles develop.

There are two major areas in which studies have proven an increased risk for postmenopausal women and protection from estrogen. The first of these is cardiovascular disease. The average woman has a 31 percent lifetime chance of dying from coronary artery heart disease, compared to 2.8 percent from breast cancer, and 2.8 percent from the results of severe osteoporotic fractures. The risk of dying from cancer of the uterus is 0.7 percent. Women tend to live longer than men, and the onset of cardiovascular disease in women is ten to twenty years later than it is in men. More women die of cardiovascular disease than of cancer, however, especially after the age of seventy. Women on estrogen replacement therapy have a lower incidence of death year by year due to coronary artery disease than do women not taking estrogen. The overall relative risk of coronary artery disease for women who have ever taken hormone replacement therapy is .65. In other words, the risk of dying at any given year is reduced by one third. For women currently taking hormone replacement therapy, the risk is .49—in other words, it is half the risk of those not taking it in any specific year of age.

Estrogen protects the coronary arteries in several ways. First, it has a positive effect on cholesterol, by reducing total cholesterol and LDL cholesterol and increasing HDL cholesterol (the protective cholesterol). The second advantage is that estrogen acts as an antioxidant and therefore has a positive effect on removing any arteriosclerotic plaques that may be developing in the coronary arteries. The third positive effect of estrogen in preventing heart disease is that it dilates the coronary arteries, allowing for better blood flow through them. In one study, HDL was found to increase 13.5 percent when women used estrogen. In the same study, LDL was found to decrease by 16 percent, and total cholesterol decreased by 6 percent.

In addition to the positive effect that estrogen therapy has on preventing heart disease, there is also evidence that it prevents stroke. A study performed at the Leisure World in California found a 70 percent reduction in mortality due to stroke in users of estrogen. A second study had similar findings.

The second area of risk in postmenopausal women is that of osteoporosis and fracture. Women not taking estrogen after menopause will lose cortical bone (spinal vertebrae) at the rate of 1 to 3 percent per year and trabecular bone (long bones of the limbs) at the rate of 2 to 5 percent per year. After maximum loss over the first few years, the rate of bone loss decreases but continues. After ten to thirty years, osteoporosis becomes serious enough to cause fractures to begin. Twenty-five to 40 percent of women will have experienced fractures by the age of seventy. By age eighty, 16 percent of women will have experienced hip fractures, which can be life threatening. Fifty percent of these women will die of complications during the first year after a hip fracture, and up to 30 percent of survivors may be disabled. Fractures of the spinal vertebrae are twice as common as hip fractures, occurring in 20 to 35 percent of women over the age of sixty. Usually this is noted on X ray, and many of these fractures are without symptoms other than possible back pain. Such fractures usually result in loss of height, some deformity, and disability.

Certain women are at higher risk for osteoporosis. These include thin women, natural blondes, women of Scandinavian background, those with a family history of osteoporosis, and those who use cigarettes and alcohol. (See Table 6.1.) The risk of osteoporosis can be blunted by beginning a good calcium intake early in life. This should be about 1,000 to 1,500 mg per day. Weight-bearing exercises are also important. Some women, among them African Americans, generally have thicker bones and therefore are less susceptible to osteoporosis. Estrogen replacement therapy slows the rate of cortical and trabecular bone reabsorption and reduces the incidence of fractures. It should be noted, however, that the aging process will continue, and the tendency for bone to demineralize, even though greatly reduced, will continue. Clearly, a ninety-year-old person will not have the bone density of a thirty-year-old person even with estrogen replacement therapy. Estrogen use slows the natural process rather than eliminating it. Nonetheless, great benefits may be derived for longevity and quality of life with estrogen use.

TABLE 6.1.   Risk Factors for Osteoporosis

Thin body build

Natural blonde

Scandinavian origin

Family history of osteoporosis

Smoker

Alcohol use

A recent report from the Leisure World study involves tooth loss. Women who used estrogen were shown to experience less tooth loss than did nonusers. Since gum disease and tooth decay do not adequately define all of the reasons for tooth loss, one theory is that it may be related to osteoporosis and that this may be partially reversed by estrogen.

SHOULD I USE ESTROGEN REPLACEMENT THERAPY?

CASE STUDY

Julie is fifty-one years old. She consulted me because she had not had a menstrual period for six months. She has been a patient of mine for a number of years, and I had only seen her on an annual basis for her health maintenance visits since the birth of her last child fifteen years ago. Her periods were never irregular. They stopped without any problems, and she has had minimal hot flashes and night sweats. She has not noted vaginal dryness, and intercourse is still comfortable. She had always enjoyed good health and has had no surgical procedures. Her three children were born vaginally and are living and well. Her mother, who is alive at age eighty, has never taken estrogen replacement therapy and is in reasonably good health. Julie is five feet, two inches tall and weighs 120 pounds. She plays tennis and golf and has a part-time job as a school librarian. She has heard many good things about hormone replacement therapy but is also frightened that it may cause her to develop cancer. Many newspaper articles and radio presentations have frightened her. She came in asking whether or not I believe she needs estrogen replacement therapy.

First of all, I explained the many benefits to estrogen therapy, but I told her that she should not take any medication she was not comfortable with. I suggested that she continue her exercise regimen, to be sure to do weight-bearing exercise (running, jogging, walking, tennis, golf, and so on) at least three times per week. I also encouraged her to take 1,500 mg of calcium per day whether or not she decided to use estrogen replacement therapy.

After having dealt with the benefits of estrogen replacement therapy, we next discussed the potential hazards. Julie has no health hazards at the present time and therefore no major contraindications to estrogen therapy. But what are the risks of cancer? First of all, there is no evidence that estrogen replacement therapy causes cancer of the vulva, vagina, cervix, fallopian tube, or ovary. Many years ago, when estrogen was first utilized for hormone replacement therapy, it was utilized in much higher doses than we use today and was not opposed by progesterone. With this unopposed high-dose estrogen therapy, popular during the 1960s and early 1970s, the risk of cancer of the uterus (endometrial cancer) increased, becoming as much as eightfold more than the incidence seen in women who were not using estrogen. But with lower dose estrogen therapy and with progesterone utilization, this increased incidence of endometrial cancer has disappeared.

What about cancer of the breast? This is a difficult one to sort out because the epidemiologic studies available to us tend to be quite variable in the way they deal with women of different age groups. By age fifty, a woman has about a 2 percent chance of getting breast cancer. This increases with each year of longevity so that by about age ninety, a woman has a 1 in 8 chance of having breast cancer. Thus, the risk increases with age, and the longer one lives, the greater the chance of breast cancer. Many of the epidemiologic studies lump women over sixty or sixty-five together. Since the incidence of cancer is going up year by year and since estrogen replacement therapy protects the heart and the bones, it is very possible that it is because the women who are using estrogen replacement therapy are living to an older age that they have a greater chance of developing breast cancer. Thus, if one lumps all women over sixty-five together, a false impression may be obtained. Another piece of good news comes from a study that looked at the risk of breast cancer in high-risk women, that is, women whose mothers or sisters had breast cancer. There was no difference in the incidence of breast cancer in these women whether or not they took estrogen. Finally, in a group of women who did develop breast cancer, those who were on estrogen therapy had a better prognosis than those who were not, perhaps implying that the estrogen modulated the lethality of the cancer in some fashion.

We do not have the data to state unequivocally that estrogen is safe and that the risk of breast cancer is no greater in estrogen users than in nonusers. But if there is an increased rate, it is probably a very small one. To date, estrogen has not been positively related to the development of any other cancers. My patient Julie decided upon the basis of this information to use estrogen replacement therapy.

Some women believe that taking estrogen will cause weight gain and eventually lead to obesity. In a recent study of women using estrogen replacement therapy long-term, performed at the University of California, San Diego, no evidence was found that estrogen was related in any way to the development of obesity. The study also found no change in fat distribution or body composition. The findings held whether the women studied used hormones continuously or intermittently. Most such changes seen with aging are due to the aging process and not to hormone therapy.

HOW IS HORMONE REPLACEMENT GIVEN?

There are many ways to give hormone replacement therapy. The therapeutically active ingredient that is responsible for the positive effects that I have described is estrogen. Progesterone is given only to protect the endometrium from developing a thickened lining (hyperplasia) or endometrial cancer. For women who have had hysterectomies, progesterone supplementation is not necessary. In fact, at least in a minor way, it may counterbalance the positive effects of estrogen on cholesterol since progesterone tends to increase total cholesterol and LDL cholesterol while reducing HDL cholesterol. Thus, a woman who has no uterus need only take estrogen, but a woman with a uterus should take progesterone as well except in some very rare instances.

Estrogen may be given in several ways. Many preparations are available for oral use. One of the most popular, which probably comprises about 70 percent of the hormone replacement therapy in the United States, is conjugated equine estrogens. This has been marketed for years under the trade name of Premarin, and it is available in several doses.

For postmenopausal women, studies have shown that the 0.625 mg daily dose produces a blood level of estrogen close to the one women experience during the time they are actually menstruating. This dose has minimal effects on liver globulins and therefore usually does not increase a woman's susceptibility to an increased risk of thrombophlebitis and resultant pulmonary embolism. Higher doses may interfere with liver globulin production, and some of these globulins, which are related to the clotting factors, may increase the risk of vascular clotting. Women seem more susceptible to this problem as they age. Younger women can tolerate higher doses of estrogen, and most birth control pills have an estrogen potency of about four times greater than 0.625 mg of Premarin. However, many younger women deprived of their ovaries or ovarian function require higher doses of Premarin to relieve the uncomfortable symptoms of hot flashes and night sweats and to protect their bones from osteoporosis. There are two other pills that should be of use for younger women; these are the 0.9 mg and 1.25 mg doses. Some older women require a dose of 0.9 mg in order to be symptom free, but it is probably unwise to go higher. In addition to the increased risk of vascular clotting, it has been shown that the maximum cholesterol effect is obtained at lower doses and is actually reversed at doses of 1.25 mg per day. Thus, the ideal dose of Premarin for women over fifty years of age is 0.625 mg.

A 0.3 mg dose of Premarin has been shown to relieve the symptoms of hot flashes and night sweats in most women. It may be a sufficient dose for small women. Studies have shown that about 80 percent of women are protected from developing osteoporosis on this dose, but the 0.625 mg protects just about 100 percent. Taking estrogen orally allows for the estrogen absorbed in the intestinal tract to be shunted through the liver before it goes to the rest of the body. Because this stimulates the cholesterol response in the liver, the oral form of estrogen may be somewhat beneficial. There are other popular forms of oral estrogen. One is Estrace, which is 17 beta-estradiol. This comes in 0.5, 1.0, and 2 mg doses, and for most women the 1 mg dose is sufficient to relieve symptoms and get the desired beneficial effects for the heart and bones. Another form is estropipate, marketed as Ogen. This comes in dosages of 0.625 mg, 1.25 mg, and 2.5 mg tablets. In general, Ogen has about half the potency of Premarin, so a dose of 1.25 mg is generally required to produce the equivalent effect of 0.625 mg of Premarin. This is, however, a useful estrogen that is well tolerated by many women. Other companies produce oral estrogens in various forms, but these three preparations are the most commonly prescribed in the United States.

The second way estrogen is commonly delivered is by transdermal patch. This allows the estrogen to be absorbed over time gradually through the skin. The oldest and most commonly used of these is Estraderm, which comes in doses 0.05 mg and 0.10 mg. These patches deliver estradiol directly to the circulation, and in general the 0.05 mg patch is equivalent to a dose of 0.625 mg of Premarin, whereas the 0.10 mg patch is equivalent to the 1.25 mg dose of Premarin. These patches need to be changed roughly every three days. Up to 25 percent of women will notice a skin reaction from the patch, but the effects of this are not harmful. Many women who enjoy the convenience of a transdermal patch will put up with the low-grade skin reaction. There are currently newer transdermal patches that utilize a different delivery system and allow for a twice or once-a-week application of the patch. These are sold under the trade names of Climara and Vivelle.

Estrogen can also be delivered by injection of a long-acting preparation that can last for about a week or can be inserted under the skin in the pellet form. In the United States most women seem to prefer the oral or transdermal forms, which are extremely adequate for the therapeutic response required.

Progesterone can also be delivered in several forms. The important thing is that progesterone be given for ten to fourteen days each month, whereas estrogen is given daily. A popular progestin for this purpose is medroxyprogesterone acetate, which is commonly marketed under the brand name Provera. The usual dosages is 5 to 10 mg per day, with a 10 mg dose being the most popular since it has been shown to be the most protective. Many women do not like the side effects of progesterone, which can include weight gain, bloating, and in as many as 10 percent of women, depression. Often hormone replacement therapy is discontinued because of the effects of progesterone.

Recently, 5 mg of Provera or an equivalent amount of a different progesterone has been used in several trials and appears to offer reasonable protection for the endometrium with respect to hyperplasia formation. Several physicians have utilized this dosage in treating their patients, with better results. Also, many physicians will treat women with progesterone every third month instead of every month. This will usually cause a menstrual flow only at the times that the progesterone compound is utilized. While patients often prefer this approach, its safety as compared to the monthly use of progesterone has not been adequately studied.

Other progestins are available for use, but all have about the same effect on the endometrium and the same side effects.

Several dosage regimens can be utilized (see Table 6.2). A common one that is popular for women during the first few years of the postmenopausal period is a daily dose of estrogen such as 0.625 mg of Premarin, 1 mg of Estrace or 1.25 mg of Ogen, and ten days per month of Provera at 5 to 10 mg daily. In most women this will allow periods to continue generally during the first few days after stopping the progesterone. Since the estrogen dose noted will only give women a blood level of estrogen equivalent to what they would have had when they were actually menstruating, it is not necessary to stop estrogen. For years it was given in a cyclic fashion, with women being told to stop all medications for 5 to 7 days per month. This is no longer necessary, but many women and doctors still utilize that regimen. There does not seem to be any benefit from doing this as compared to using daily estrogen. The cyclic method of dosing with estrogen and progesterone is especially good for women who are just past menopause, as ovarian function probably continues for up to three years. Up to 30 to 40 percent of women who try using a daily regimen of estrogen and progesterone immediately after menopause will have breakthrough bleeding, which can be worrisome and annoying. In women who are three or more years past menopause, a daily regimen of estrogen as noted (that is, Premarin 0.625 mg per day), with a low dose of Provera such as 2.5 mg or 5 mg every day, will get the beneficial effects desired but generally without any breakthrough bleeding or menstrual periods. Many women begin with a cyclic regimen and then later switch to a daily combined regimen. There are now available daily doses of estrogen replacement therapy that contain both estrogen and progesterone for this purpose. One popular combination is marketed as Prempro.

TABLE 6.2.   Dosage Schedule for Hormone Replacement

Regimen	Schedule
1.	Estrogen daily, progesterone 10–14 days each month
2.	Estrogen daily, progesterone daily (lower dose)
3.	Estrogen daily 1–25 each calendar month, progesterone day 16–25
4.	Estrogen 5 days out of 7

In occasional cases, women cannot tolerate progesterone and therefore would not use hormone replacement therapy. Experience in Europe and in several practices in the United States has demonstrated that low doses of estrogen may be safely given five days out of seven without progesterone. Women who wish to do this must realize that they are taking the medication outside the usual and customary way it is prescribed and should have either an endometrial biopsy or an ultrasound examination measuring the thickness of the endometrial lining annually. In general, if the endometrial lining is found on ultrasound to be 5 mm or less in thickness there is probably no risk that hyperplasia or endometrial cancer is developing. If the lining is noted to be thicker than 5 to 8 mm, an endometrial biopsy is performed. It is equally useful but not nearly as comfortable to perform an endometrial biopsy annually. Women who subscribe to the estrogen-only regimen and have intact uteruses should be followed closely with this annual surveillance. If you cannot tolerate progesterone, this is something you might discuss with your doctor to see whether or not it is reasonable alternative for you. Also, it is important to emphasize at this point that any women on an estrogen replacement therapy regimen, no matter what it may be, who bleeds abnormally should be given an endometrial biopsy to be sure that hyperplasia or cancer is not developing. In the past, a D&C would be performed, but we now have techniques for removing a small sample as an office procedure that is just about as effective as a complete dilatation and curettage under anesthesia and certainly much more cost effective and comfortable.

CONTRAINDICATIONS TO HORMONE REPLACEMENT THERAPY

There are several contraindications to estrogen use. Currently, women who have had either breast or endometrial cancer are generally not given hormone replacement therapy. There is no strong data that estrogen causes breast cancer, but we do have some data indicating that it is associated with an increase in endometrial cancer when given without progesterone or in high doses. The question of whether or not a woman could eventually take hormone replacement therapy after she has recovered from either breast or uterine cancer has not yet been answered. Several physicians are offering hormone replacement therapy to women who have had breast cancer if the breast cancer was small with negative lymph nodes and if it has been more than five years since therapy. Again, this is outside the usual bounds of customary therapy, and a woman considering it should discuss this carefully with her physician before undertaking such a plan. It is less clear whether or not women who have had endometrial cancer should use hormone replacement therapy, but probably if they have had an early well-differentiated tumor removed more than five years ago, it may be safe for them to use it. The data to support this are not available, and the woman and her physician must weigh the woman's symptoms and risk for other diseases against whatever small risk may exist for using hormone therapy.

Women with liver disease should probably not use hormone replacement therapy, as these steroid hormones are detoxified in the liver. If the liver cannot adequately detoxify them, they will build up in the blood and make the woman more susceptible to endometrial and possibly breast cancer.

Some women suffer from hypertension, which seems to be aggravated by estrogen. They should be thoroughly evaluated by a physician and probably should not be given hormone replacement therapy. On the other hand, most women with hypertension can tolerate hormone therapy once their hypertension is adequately treated.

Another contraindication may be a history of thrombophlebitis or pulmonary embolism related to pregnancy or to the use of oral contraceptives. Although the dosage schedules used for hormone replacement therapy are such that liver globulins that affect coagulation are usually not elevated, some woman may have a hereditary defect affecting their clotting mechanism that may be aggravated by estrogen. There are several such defects, and not all of them contraindicate the use of estrogen. Again, a physician should be consulted and the woman thoroughly evaluated before a decision is made.

Although there is a relationship between smokers over the age thirty-five, oral contraceptive use, and heart disease, the same relationship does not seem to be present in estrogen replacement therapy users who smoke. Smoking, of course, increases the risk of many illnesses for patients. Women should stop smoking rather than do without hormone replacement therapy and its benefits.

Other Medications

While estrogen is the surest way of reducing the complaints of hot flashes and night sweats, there are a few other medications that may be useful for the woman who cannot take estrogen. Progesterone in small doses will alleviate these symptoms, at least in part, in about 80 percent of patients. Therefore, women who have had breast cancer and do not wish to take estrogen may be able to take progesterone and get relief.

A preparation called Clonidine has been demonstrated in studies to significantly reduce the number of hot flashes. This medication can be given via transdermal patch, but it does have an effect of raising blood pressure in some women. It should therefore be used with the close supervision of a physician. In rare cases, it may interfere with the electrical conduction of the heart and mimic the circumstances under which patients have been prescribed cardiac pacemakers. In a woman who is otherwise healthy and is bothered by hot flashes and night sweats and is unable to take estrogen, however, this is often a reasonable alternative.

With respect to preventing osteoporosis, there is a group of medications called bis-phosphonates. These are not a replacement for estrogen, but they do have a direct effect on bone. One bisphosphonate that was recently introduced after extensive clinical trial is known as Fosamax. In a study of a large group of women, half of whom were given Fosamax and the other half a placebo, 3.2 percent of those on Fosamax suffered vertebral fractures, compared to 6.2 percent on placebo. When measured on the yearly basis, there was a 63 percent reduction in the number of new vertebral fractures in the Fosamax group and 35 percent less height loss. There seemed to be a significant increase in bone density in those on the drug, as compared to those taking the placebo. The medication has to be given very carefully. It should be taken with water in the morning on an empty stomach and while sitting up. No food or other medications should be put into the stomach for at least half an hour so that absorption is ensured. While the medication is generally well tolerated, there have been reports of irritation of the upper gastrointestinal tract, including the esophagus and the stomach. On the other hand, these are common general complaints, and several patients on the placebo group also complained of them. This medications seems to help build bone rather than merely prevent demineralization and offer some hope for the future for people with osteoporosis. It is likely that other new medications of this type will be developed.

Calcium supplementation in a dose of about 1,500 mg per day is important for all women, as is weight-bearing exercise. Calcium and weight-bearing exercises in and of themselves will not significantly reduce fractures, but they will probably help to slow the demineralization process.

Some physicians and patients believe that male sex hormones (androgens) may be helpful in certain situations to help increase patient energy level and to improve sexual libido. The ovaries continue to produce androgen after menopause, and women with intact ovaries probably do not need supplementation. Women who have had their ovaries surgically removed and are suffering from decreased sexual interest, and generally decreased energy, may benefit by some androgen supplementation. There is not a great deal of scientific data to prove this point one way or the other, and it is not the general feeling that all women should be given androgens. There are some preparations that combine estrogen and natural testosterone and can be taken as a single daily pill. One of these, Estratest, contains conjugated equine estrogen with methyl testosterone. In general, testosterone elevates the total cholesterol and LDL cholesterol and therefore may, to a certain extent, counteract the beneficial effects on cholesterol of estrogen. For a woman for whom this medication may seem indicated, the physician will need to weight the risks versus the potential benefits, in consultation with her.

THE ESTROGEN JUNKIE

Menopause is very difficult transitional time for some women. It is a time when children are finally out of the home and both spouses may be going through both health and social changes. Therefore, depression and other psychosocial stresses may come into play at about the same time. Estrogen is a mood elevator and does make many women feel better. Unfortunately, as with most other medications, tolerance is rapidly developed, and in order to maintain mood elevation, higher doses of estrogen are continuously required. Thus, some women seek more and more estrogen in the belief that their metabolism is different from those of other women and that they require more estrogen to get the desired results. Often physicians are lured into this misunderstanding and will indeed prescribe larger doses of estrogen. Women with uteruses are of course at risk for developing hyperplasia and cancer as megadoses of estrogen are prescribed. Since they may be depressed, and progesterone may make the symptoms worse, the tendency is for many women not to take progesterone supplementation, thereby increasing the risk of hyperplasia and cancer.

CASE STUDY

Edith is a fifty-five-year-old woman married to a prominent minister. She went through menopause at age fifty, she has three grown children, all of whom are healthy and she participates actively in the affairs of her church and community. At the time of her menopause she was placed on hormone replacement therapy consisting of Premarin .625 mg daily and Provera 10 mg for ten days per month. She continued to have periods but after a short time began experiencing hot flashes, night sweats, and a fair amount of nervousness and depression, as she had before therapy. She discussed this with her physician, who increased the dose of Premarin to .9 mg and later to 1.2 mg per day. She would feel better for a few weeks to a month, and then the same symptoms would return. On her own, she doubled the dose of estrogen and was taking 2.5 mg per day along with her usual dose of progesterone. Again she experienced some relief for a few months, followed by a return of her symptoms. She consulted another physician and was given the impression that perhaps her metabolism was more active than that of most women, possibly because she was more active. This physician prescribed estrogen injections, and she took one every week. She noticed that she would feel well for a few days, but by the end of the week, her symptoms had returned. Her physician became perplexed with the lack of response and referred her to me for consultation. She was generally in good health but was obviously a nervous woman who had a good deal of anxiety about why she was not responding to the estrogen doses she was taking. She stated that she had heard about implantation of estrogen pellets and wondered if I thought this would be a good idea.

After taking a complete history from Edith, I ascertained that she did indeed have several of the symptoms of depression. She would fall asleep at night but wake up in two hours and then be up for the rest of the night. Her appetite was poor, and she had lost about ten pounds. She stated that she got very little pleasure out of any of her daily activities and was strongly looking forward to a time when her husband would retire from his pastoral duties, although he enjoyed these and showed no indication of planning for such an event. I prescribed for her a mild antidepressant and gradually reduced her dose of estrogen. She required the antidepressant therapy for about a year and then was able to stop its use. Currently, she is using Premarin .625 mg daily and Provera 10 mg for ten days out of each month.

Mild depression is quite common in up to 20 percent of Americans at some time during their lives. They may certainly experience it more than once, but therapy does not necessarily have to be continued forever. Depression is common at times of transition, and menopause certainly qualifies as one of those times. Edith was getting benefits from the mood elevation of the estrogen, but estrogen is not a good antidepressant over the long haul. Her case is not at all unique. I probably see one or two patients a month with similar stories in my referral practice. Being mildly depressed at various times in one's life is not a sign of mental illness or failure, and it should be looked upon as any other illness and treated accordingly. Estrogen is an excellent therapy for the menopause, but it should not be abused.

CONCLUSION

The menopause is really a time of the failure of an organ, namely the ovary. If it is viewed as a hormonal deficiency syndrome, then it makes perfect sense to use replacement hormone therapy to alleviate the symptoms and the progressive nature of this deficiency. It is reasonable, however, for women to make the choice themselves as to whether or not they will use hormone replacement therapy. The choice should be made with full knowledge of the benefits and potential risks. Certainly, this choice should be made after consultation with each woman's physician, who knows her situation best. No medication should be taken in fear; women who are not convinced that this is an appropriate course of action for them should make their own decision, preferably with the guidance of their physician.

The benefits of hormone replacement therapy are many, and the risks are probably very few. It is very likely that a woman's life will be extended and enhanced by the use of these medications. If a woman is not going to use estrogen replacement therapy, then she should be monitored very carefully for the developing signs of osteoporosis and heart disease, so that other medications can be utilized early. Certainly all women should use calcium and engage in weight-bearing exercise.

The menopause is a transitional time of life, but most women have one third of their lives ahead of them after they pass through this time. It is the responsibility of both the woman and her physician to use every means at their disposal to ensure that this will be a comfortable, happy, and productive time.

CHAPTER 7

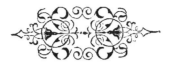

Immunizations and Travel Health Concerns

Proper immunization provides protection against many infectious diseases that can cause death or disability, and it usually acts with very little risk of any serious health hazard. Most of us received a battery of these immunizations as young children, and during the past several decades immunization has been given for smallpox, diphtheria, tetanus, pertussis (whopping cough), polio, and, more recently, rubella (German measles), measles (red measles), and mumps. Very recently pediatricians have been recommending that all children be given hepatitis B immunization. This chapter describes the routine immunizations that everyone should receive as well as special cases that may require additional immunization.

ROUTINE IMMUNIZATIONS FOR OLDER WOMEN

You probably received immunization against tetanus, diphtheria, and whooping cough as a child. Because of this universal immunization program, which has been in effect in the United States for many years, tetanus and diphtheria are very rare diseases. But immunizations may not be protective for a lifetime, and booster shots are necessary. The Centers for Disease Control recommend a booster shot for tetanus and diphtheria every ten years. Your health professional will probably keep a record of when you receive these in your health chart, but it is worthwhile for you to obtain a yellow immunization card and keep track of these shots yourself. If you keep this immunization up, you will not have to worry about getting tetanus if you step on a rusty nail, are bitten by a dog, or have some other injury that conceivably could introduce tetanus bacteria into your system. Also, if you become exposed to diphtheria, you will not be infected by it.

The Centers for Disease Control also recommend annual influenza vaccine shots beginning at age sixty-five. As people age, bronchial trees become more rigid and mucus movement is reduced. For someone who contracts viral influenza, damage to the bronchial tree may be such that bacterial secondary infections take place. This can lead to pneumonia, and with it there is a risk of mortality. Thus, protection against influenza is particularly important in older people. Although the CDC suggest that annual immunization begin at age sixty-five, I generally recommend them for my patients over sixty. In some high-risk situations, people should receive immunization at an even earlier age.

Along the same lines, there is currently a recommendation that pneumococcal vaccine be given in one dose after the age of sixty-five. For the same reasons as those that pertain to influenza, the increasing rigidity of the bronchial tree makes people more susceptible to bacterial pneumonia. Vaccination against the pneumonococcus, the most common cause of bacterial pneumonia, is reasonable. Although it is still controversial whether or not this actually significantly prevents pneumonia, most physicians now agree that it is worth giving to their older patients and that it probably should be repeated every six to seven years. The minimum routine immunizations for older individuals are summarized in Table 7.1.

IMMUNIZATION IN HIGH-RISK SITUATIONS

If you never received tetanus and diphtheria vaccine, you should be immunized against them with a three-dose schedule. The pediatric vaccine that contains whooping cough (pertussis toxoid) is not necessary for adults, since they have either had the disease or been exposed to it. Following the initial vaccination, a booster schedule of every ten years should be instituted.

Since polio has been pretty much eradicated in the United States, routine primary or booster immunization for adults who are not leaving the country is not deemed necessary at the present time. There are, however, certain risk situations. For instance, adults who have not been immunized or whose immunization may have waned could be at a small risk for developing paralytic polio from the stool of a child who has recently been given the live virus oral polio vaccine. Thus, parents, grandparents, or day care workers who may be in contact with such children should be given either a booster immunization or the full three-dose primary vaccination schedule if they have never been vaccinated. Adults planning to travel to areas where polio is endemic should also be immunized. Adults who suffer from immunodeficiency virus (HIV) or

TABLE 7.1.   Minimum Routine Immunizations

Immunizations	Schedule
Tetanus-diphtheria booster (TD)	Every 10 years
Influenza vaccine	Annually at age 60–65
Pneumococcal vaccine	One dose at or about age 65, repeated every 6–7 years

other immunodeficiencies should not be given live polio vaccine but should use the inactivated polio virus. Although vaccine-associated polio is rare, it is more common in adults than in children. It is suggested that adults receiving primary immunization should be given the inactivated form known as e-IPV. It is produced on cultured human cells with the antibiotic streptomycin added. Adults who have a history of sensitivity to this antibiotic should not receive this vaccine.

Although most adults have either been immunized against measles, mumps, and German measles (rubella) or have had the diseases, those who have not may wish to be immunized. Measles and mumps outbreaks seem to be sporadic, but they may occur, and they carry a risk of mortality and disability when they infect older people. Those who have not been vaccinated and who are traveling to endemic areas should consider the vaccination. The vaccine is made from live but attenuated virus administered in two doses. Currently it is suggested that people born before 1957 have probably had clinical or subclinical cases and probably do not need vaccination. Those traveling to endemic areas or who work as health care workers, particularly if they were born after 1957, should be immunized. Anyone who was been immunized prior to 1957 should probably be given a second dose, as the vaccine has been improved. The vaccine is produced on chicken embryo cells with neomycin antibiotic added. Anyone who is allergic to eggs or neomycin should not receive this vaccine.

Health care workers who are exposed to many patients should be immunized against hepatitis B and should be given annual flu vaccines. People with chronic diseases, particularly respiratory diseases, should be given annual flu vaccine and the pnuomococcal vaccine. Residents in chronic care facilities should receive annual flu vaccine. People who are immunodeficient, which includes patients with HIV infection, those who have received organ transplants, and those who have had their spleens removed should receive the pneumococcal vaccine. People who may come in contact with blood or blood products, such as IV drug abusers, dialysis recipients, and those who receive blood products for other reasons should be immunized against hepatitis B. (See Table 7.2.)

TABLE 7.2.   Indications for Hepatitis B Immunization

Health Risk Group	Immunization Recommendation
Health care worker	Hepatitis B, annual flu vaccine
Chronic diseases (especially respiratory conditions)	Annual flu vaccine; pneumococcal vaccine
Residents of chronic care facilities	Annual flu vaccine
Immunodeficient individuals	Pneumococcal vaccine
Individuals exposed to blood or blood products	Hepatitis B

Recently hepatitis A vaccine has become available. Hepatitis A is the infectious hepatitis that is contracted from contaminated food or contact with individuals who are infected with the virus. People have frequently contracted this at fast food restaurants from a food handler who has been found to have the disease or from contaminated food such as raw oysters. Hepatitis A can leave the sufferer extremely sick with jaundice, which can leave the liver permanently damaged. In the past, anyone exposed to this condition was given a dose of gamma globulin obtained from the blood of patients recovering from this disease. This gave protection for up to three months. Gamma globulin was also given to people who were traveling to areas endemic for hepatitis A. The protection was again good for about three months, meaning that every time the person was at risk, gamma globulin was necessary. Recently, a vaccine has been developed for hepatitis A that is administered in a two-dose schedule with a six-month interval between shots. It is worthwhile for everyone to receive this vaccination. Currently, it is the practice of most physician offices and clinics to give the first shot of vaccine, rather than using gamma globulin, to people who have been exposed. This seems to give as much protection as a gamma globulin shot. The second shot of the series can be given six months later. Certainly people who travel to endemic areas or areas whose sanitation is poor, or who may be in contact with people with hepatitis A, should receive the vaccination.

There are contraindications to immunizations, and these are summarized in Table 7.3.

TABLE 7.3.   Contraindications for Specific Immunizations

Immunization	Contraindication
All immunizations	Allergic reaction to previous administration
	Allergic reaction to a vaccine constinuent
	Moderate to severe illness (with or without a fever)
Oral polio (OPV)	HIV infection, household contact with HIV, other immunodeficiency conditions
Inactive polio vaccine (IPV)	Anaphylactic reaction to neomycin or streptomycin
Measles, mumps, rubella (MMR)	Anaphylactic reaction to egg ingestion or neomycin; pregnancy; immunodeficiency
Hepatitis B	None identified
Hepatitis A	None identified
Influenza	Anphylactic reaction to eggs

TRAVEL IMMUNIZATIONS AND PROPHYLAXES

If you are traveling outside the United States, it is best to determine what diseases you may be exposed to and what prophylaxes against disease may be necessary. Advice you may need can be obtained from your physician, a travel clinic, or from contacting the Centers for Disease Control in Atlanta, Georgia. The CDC will either send or fax you information pertaining to the areas you plan to visit. Their telephone number is (404)-639-1610.

Malaria is still a major problem throughout the world and is endemic in Central America, South America, Africa, India, and Asia. There are several different types of malaria, and some are resistant to the common prophylactic agents, such as chloroquine, that have been used in the past. Resistant forms require newer and in many cases somewhat toxic agents. Since this is a rapidly changing field, it is important to discuss your needs with your travel clinic or to utilize the information from the CDC to determine which agent best suits your purpose. Malaria is a potentially lethal or crippling disease and should be avoided. Therefore, appropriate prophylaxes should be utilized.

CHAPTER 8

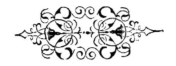

Sexuality: How to Use It and Not Lose It

Sexuality is a behavioral phenomenon that is influenced by many factors. The health and physiologic state of each person is important, and so is the importance that the person has placed on sexual activity as a source of comfort and gratification in earlier life. As a behavior it is strongly influenced by the people and associations that are part of the person's life. While advancing age is almost always associated with a decrease in sexual function and satisfaction, failing health and many medications may also contribute.

In a study of more than four thousand adults over age fifty, most individuals stated that they were still sexually active, and those who were reported happier marriages and relationships than did sexually inactive counterparts of similar age. In this study, women showed a more marked decline than did men in the desire to remain sexually active. Masturbation as a form of sexual gratification remained stable in women but gradually declined in men with age. Other studies have demonstrated that women past menopause often note a decreasing sexual desire and orgasmic response. Not all women respond in the same fashion, however, and in a study of perimenopausal and postmenopausal women, 49 percent reported a decline in sexual activity with the change or cessation of menses, 38 percent reported no change, and 14 percent actually reported increased interest. In the very old, intercourse is often less likely with advancing age, but the frequency of caressing behavior remains. Several elderly men and women in the study reported increased interest in caressing and masturbation but decreasing interest in intercourse.

Women's sexual interest and responses often are related to the abilities of their partner, relating as much to the health and vigor of the partner as to the health and vigor of the woman herself. Women who have good marriages generally have greater satisfaction in their sexual relationships. Although psychiatric factors and gynecologic problems are, for the most part, unrelated to sexual behavior, women who suffer from depression frequently note decreased sexual satisfaction.

After menopause, the levels of estrogen and progesterone are reduced. This is the case even in women on hormone replacement therapy. Testosterone levels may also be reduced. The thickness and elasticity of the vaginal and urinary tracts are decreased, as is the amount of vaginal lubrication. The acidity of the vagina usually decreases, and the woman may be susceptible to vaginal irritation and low-grade infection. From a physiologic standpoint, there is generally an increase in the amount of time necessary for sexual arousal and a decrease in the number and intensity of orgasmic contractions. With aging and the postmenopausal period, there is generally a loss of elasticity and smoothness of facial and body skin, which may be perceived as a loss of attractiveness and thus may contribute to a decrease in sexual interest in the couple in some cases. There is also a greater likelihood of illness and the need for medication in this age group, which may affect many of the aspects of sexual response. To some extent, hormone replacement therapy prevents some of these changes.

On the psychosocial side, many influences may be in play. Cultural stereotypes of older people include the perception that they may be desexualized or unattractive. Society, in some cases, views sexuality in women beyond the childbearing years suspiciously. In certain societies, the cultural definition of sexuality for older women may be so narrow that the woman herself may see her sexual desires as abnormal.

Older women may also suffer a decreased availability of males for relationships, since women often outlive their male counterparts or may be partnered with a male who is experiencing sexual problems because of his own health and aging process. Older women often suffer many losses, which lead to grief reactions, which may limit the amount of emotional energy available for sexual activity.

Finally, genital appearance may change, especially due to lack of estrogen, leading to thinning and dryness of the vaginal epithelium, decreased fullness of the clitoris and labia, and a reduction of pubic hair. The vagina may shrink in length and become narrow in diameter, and if intercourse is not practiced for long periods of time, it may actually close. The atrophy of the vaginal tissues that are involved in these changes increases the susceptibility to vaginal infections, vaginal tears, and other irritations. These factors, in and of themselves, may convince a woman to avoid intercourse.

Sexual function is under the influence of the involuntary (autonomic) nervous system. There are two components to this: the sympathetic and the parasympathetic nervous systems. The nerve junctions of the parasympathetic system depend upon the neurotransmitter, acetyl choline. The nerve junctions of the sympathetic system depend on the neurotransmitter, norepinephrine. The autonomic nervous system is involved in many bodily functions, including the regulation of blood pressure, heart rate, the respiratory system, the gastrointestinal system, and kidney function. Since many of the problems of aging involve these systems, it is not surprising that medications designed to counteract the symptoms of diseases of these organ systems could have an associated effect on sexuality. The parasympathetic nervous system is necessary for arousal. It allows for vascular engorgement of the sexual organs and the breasts. In a woman, it increases the length and thickness of the clitoris, engorges the labia, and allows for an increased vaginal secretion. In a man, it allows for an erection. Along with the physiologic aspects of arousal, this nervous system reaction also allows for an increase in the psychic phenomenon of desire. The parasympathetic nervous system can be thought of as the portion of the nervous system involved in the seduction and arousal aspect of sexual activity. Thus, medications that interfere with this system may be responsible for a reduction in sexual desire and arousal response. Many tranquilizers and blood pressure medications, as well as several of the medications used to regulate digestive activities, fall into this category.

The sympathetic nervous system is responsible for orgasm, so medications that affect the sympathetic nervous system may interfere with the normal process leading to an orgasmic response. While orgasm may occur, it may not be with the customary intensity. In medicated people, it is not uncommon to see arousal take place normally but orgasm not be possible, or arousal problems may be overcome by repetitive sexual behavior, but orgasm may occur normally. Table 8-1 lists some commonly used medications and their potential effects on sexual response.

TABLE 8.1.   Drugs That May Affect Sexual Function

Drug	Adverse Effect
Acetazolamide (Diamox and others)	Loss of libido; decreased potency
Alprazolam (Xanax)	Inhibition of orgasm; delayed or no ejaculation
Amiloride (Midamor)	Impotence; decreased libido
Amiodarone (Cordarone)	Decreased libido
Amitriptyline (Elavil and others)	Loss of libido; impotence; no ejaculation
Amoxapine (Ascendin)	Loss of libido; impotence; retrograde, painful, or no ejaculation
Amphetamines and related anorexic drugs	Chronic abuse; impotence; delayed or no ejaculation in men; no orgasm in women
Anticholinergics	Impotence
Atenolol (Tenormin)	Impotence
Baclofen (Lioresal)	Impotence; inability to ejaculate
Barbiturates	Decreased libido; impotence
Carbamazepine (Tegretol)	Impotence
Chlorpromazine (Thorazine and others)	Decreased libido; impotence; no ejaculation; priapism
Chlorprothixene (Taractan)	Inhibition of ejaculation; decreased intensity of orgasm
Chlorthalidone (Hygroton and others)	Decresed libido; impotence
Cimetidine (Tagamet)	Decreased libido (men and women); impotence
Clofibrate (Atromid-S)	Decreased libido; impotence

(continued)

TABLE 8.1   *(Continued)*

Drug	Adverse Affect
Clomipramine (Anafranil)	Decreased libido; impotence; retarded or no ejaculation (men) or orgasm (women); spontaneous orgasm associated with yawning
Clonidine (Catapres and others)	Impotence; delayed or retrograde ejaculation; inhibition of orgasm (women)
Danazol (Danocrine)	Increased or decreased libido
Desipramine (Norpramin and others)	Decreased libido; impotence; difficult ejaculation and painful orgasm
Diazepam (Valium and others)	Decreased libido; delayed ejaculation; retarded or no orgasms in women
Dichlorphenamide (Daranide and others)	Decreased libido; impotence
Digoxin	Decresaed libido; impotence
Disopyramide (Norpace and others)	Impotence
Disulfiram (Antabuse and others)	Impotence
Doxepin (Adapin, Sinequan)	Decresaed libido; ejaculatory dysfunction
Estrogens	Decreased libido in men
Ethionamide (Trecator-SC)	Impotence
Ethosuximide (Zarontin)	Decreased libido
Ethoxzolamide (Ethamide)	Decreased libido
Fenfluramine (Pondimin)	Loss of libido (frequent in women with large doses or long-term use); impotence
Fluphenazine (Prolixin, Permitil)	Changes in libido; erection difficulties; inhibition of ejaculation
Guanabenz (Wytensin)	Impotence
Guanadrel (Hylorel)	Decreased libido; delayed or retrograde ejaculation; impotence
Guanethidine (Ismelin)	Decerase libido; impotence; delayed, retrograde, or no ejaculation
Guanfacine (Tenex)	Impotence
Haloperidol (Haldol and others)	Impotence; painful ejaculation
Hydralazine (Apresoline and ohters)	Impotence; priapism
Hydroxyprogesterone caporate (Delalutin and others)	Impotence

TABLE 8.1   *(Continued)*

Drug	Adverse Affect
Imipramine (Tofranil and others)	Decreased libido; impotence; painful, delayed ejaculation; delayed orgasm in women
Indapamide (Lozol)	Decreased libido; impotence
Interferon (Roferon-a)	Decreased libido; impotence
Isocarboxazid (Marplan)	Impotence; delayed ejaculation; no orgasm (women)
Ketoconazole (Nizoral)	Impotence
Lebetalol (Trandate, Normodyne)	Priapism; impotence; delayed or no ejaculation; decreased libido
Levodopa (Dopar and others)	Decreased libido; impotence
Lithium (Eskalith and others)	Decreased libido; impotence
Maprotiline (Ludiomil)	Impotence; decreased libido
Mazindol (Sanorex/Mazanor)	Impotence; spontaneous ejaculation; painful testes
Mecamylamine (Inversine)	Impotence; decreased libido
Mepenzolate bromide (Cantil)	Impotence
Mesoridazine (Serentil)	No ejaculation; impotence; priapism
Methadone (Dolophine and others)	Decreased libido; impotence; no orgasm (men and women); retarded ejaculation
Methandrostenolone (Dianobol)	Decreased libido
Mathantheline bromide (Banthine)	Impotence
Methazolamide (Neptazane)	Decreased libido (men and women); impotence; delayed or no ejaculation (men) or orgasm (women)
Methyldopa (Aldomet and others)	Decreased libido; impotence; delayed or no ejaculation (men) and orgasm (women)
Metoclopramide (Reglan and others)	Impotence; decreased libido
Metoprolol (Lopressor)	Decreased libido; impotence
Metyrosine (Demser)	Impotence; failure of ejaculation
Mexiletine (Mexitil)	Impotence; decreased libido
Molindone (Moban)	Priapism
Naltrexone (Trexan)	Delayed ejaculation; decreased potency
Naproxen (Anaprox, Naprosyn)	Impotence, no ejaculation

(continued)

TABLE 8.1   *(Continued)*

Drug	Adverse Affect
Norethindrone (Norlutin and others)	Decreased libido; impotence
Nortriptyline (Aventyl, Pamelor)	Impotence; decreased libido
Pargyline (Eutonyl)	No ejaculation; impotence
Perphenazine (Trilafon)	Decresaed or no ejaculation
Phenelzine (Nardil)	Impotence; retarded or no ejaculation; delayed or no orgasm (men and women)
Phenytoin (Dilantin and others)	Decreased libido; impotence
Pimozide (Orap)	Impotence; no ejaculation; decreased libido
Pindolol (Visken)	Impotence
Prazosin (Minipress)	Impotence; priapism
Primidone (Mysoline and others)	Decreased libido; impotence
Progesterone	Decrease libido; impotence
Propantheline bromide (Pro-Banthine and others)	Impotence
Propranolol (Inderal and others)	Loss of libido; impotence
Protriptyline (Vivactil)	Loss of libido; impotence; painful ejaculation
Ranitidine (Zantac)	Loss of libido; impotence
Reserpine	Decreased libido; impotence; decreased or no ejaculation
Spironolactone (Aldactone and others)	Decreased libido; impotence
Thiazine diuretics	Impotence
Thioridazine (Mellaril and others)	Impotence; priapism; delayed, decreased, painful, retrograde, or no ejaculation
Thiothixene (Navane and others)	Spontaneous ejaculations; impotence; priapism
Timolol (Blocadren, Timolide, Timoptic)	Decresaed libido; impotence
Tranylcypromine (Parnate)	Impotence
Trazadone (Desyrel)	Priapism; incresaed libido (women); retrograde ejaculation
Trifluoperazine (Stelazine and others)	Decreased, painful, or no ejaculation, spontaneous ejaculations
Verapamil (Calan and others)	Impotence

DIAGNOSING AND TREATING A SEXUAL PROBLEM

Many people are reluctant to discuss sexual problems. The reasons for this are many. Some may be embarrassed to bring the topic up with anyone, even a physician or partner. Often a woman may feel she is the only one to whom this is happening and thus tends to accept her fate. Although medical training in the past has not emphasized sexuality or sexual behavior, more recently there has been a tendency to try to educate physicians more fully in these areas. Still, many physicians may be neglecting to bring up the subject with their patients. If the patients are also reluctant, the matter may not be addressed. If you are having problems relating to your sexual behavior, you should indeed bring these to the attention of your physician, who may not wish to treat these but can give referrals to a health care worker who can.

The first common sexual problem is sexual desire disorders. These are quite common in older people and are defined as the persistent absence of sexual feeling or desire for sexual activity. Some women have a persistent or recurrent aversion to genital contact with a sexual partner. It is important for the health care worker and the woman to determine whether or not this is a problem of recent origin or whether the woman has always had a low sexual desire. Every individual has a different degree of libido. Many women may have strong sexual energy, whereas others may not. If the problem has been lifelong, it will be difficult to change at an advanced age. If the problem is new, it is important to sort out the reasons, since many of them can be dealt with. Clearly, a woman taking medications that interfere with the parasympathetic nervous systems will note a decrease in sexual desire. Discussing this with the physician who prescribed the medications may bring to light the possibility of changing medications to those with a less profound effect on the nervous system.

CASE STUDY

Sue Ellen, age fifty-seven, was happily married to a sixty-one-year-old orthopedist. The couple had six children, no financial problems, and a very comfortable relationship. On an annual health evaluation, Sue's husband, John, was found to have fairly severe high blood pressure and was prescribed propanolol (Inderal) by his internist. He rapidly noted loss of libido and developed impotence. The couple had always enjoyed good sexual relations, and at first both believed the problem was due to fatigue and the effects of the high blood pressure. But on a subsequent visit, when John's blood pressure was found to be normal, fortunately he discussed his problem with his doctor. His internist seemed surprised that the couple was still sexually active, but he did switch John to a different medication, and John's sexual desire and ability returned.

This couple's problem was quickly solved because John was sophisticated enough to discuss the matter with his physician. Sadly, most men are embarrassed to bring the subject up, and the couple is thus deprived of a very important activity. Occasionally, if they do not communicate with each other, the woman may blame the lack of sexual activity on herself, believing that she is no longer appealing or that her husband is having an affair with another woman.

A second major sexual problem comes from relationship problems. If the partner has undergone life changes and is no longer appealing, perhaps because of the results of an injury or a surgical procedure, or because of a chronic alcohol condition or a decrease in hygiene, the other partner may respond by having a decreased sexual desire. This may also occur if the couple's relationship is already poor or if there is abuse or intimidation. Finally, if the woman has begun to develop vaginal atrophy and intercourse is painful, this may cause a decrease in desire.

Another condition, sexual arousal disorder, is somewhat related to this. Usually in this situation there is a lack of physical response to sexual stimulation. This lack of response may be seen in the fact that there is no genital lubrication or vascular congestion. Although this may occur more prominently with advancing age, it can often be modulated with hormone therapy prescribed either vaginally or orally.

If a woman states that she would like to have intercourse but suffers from a sexual desire disorder or difficulty with arousal and has no obvious physical or psychological problem impeding this, the couple should be encouraged to increase the sexual stimulation beyond what has been their usual practice. Visual aids in the form of erotic movies or pictures are sometimes helpful. Long periods of caressing, petting, massage with fragrant oils, and so on, are often helpful. The partners should discuss openly their desires and fantasies and, whenever possible, try to satisfy them.

Orgasm problems may be a delay or absence of orgasm. The absence of orgasm during intercourse occurs in many otherwise normal couples, and it is important to determine whether or not a woman can have an orgasm by nonintercourse means such as masturbation or digital stimulation of her genitalia by her partner. It is important to determine whether or not she is taking medications that can interfere with orgasm or whether or not she suffers from illnesses that may interfere with the sympathetic nervous system. Multiple sclerosis, certain types of diabetes, and vascular diseases that involve the spinal cord may all contribute. In women who are capable of orgasm but note delay or occasional absence of orgasm, the utilization of measures that supplement intercourse are appropriate. The use of vibrators during intercourse may increase the stimulation to allow orgasm, or continued digital stimulation of the genital organs after male orgasm may allow the female partner to experience orgasm as well.

Sexual pain disorders are frequent in older women. The medical term *dyspareunia* is used when there is recurrent genital pain before, during, or after intercourse. The commonest of this in women is vaginismus. It is described as the involuntary spasm of the muscles that surround the vagina. This may occur during coitus or prior to it, preventing coitus altogether. Often it is brought about because of an injury or infection in the vagina that leads to pain with intercourse. Therefore, alleviating the cause is the most important part of therapy. Once this is done, if the spasm continues, the couple should be introduced to a plan to desensitize the woman from this response. This is relatively simple to accomplish if the cause of the pain has been removed. The woman is instructed to gently dilate her vagina with one, two, and three fingers, usually in a warm bath with total privacy ensured and often with relaxing music and fragrant soaps to improve the mood. When she has been able to dilate her vagina to two or three fingers in diameter, she may transfer this activity to her partner. At first, the couple should be instructed not to have intercourse but rather to experience caressing, petting, and digital dilation of the vagina by the partner. When this is accomplished, intercourse will usually be possible. In rare circumstances, for an older woman whose vagina has narrowed and the epithelium thinned out, it may be necessary to use vaginal estrogen treatments to improve the health of the epithelium and to use a plastic dilator to increase the width of the vagina. This, of course, should be managed under the care of a physician.

It should be mentioned that sexual satisfaction does not necessarily depend on these factors. Patients may be satisfied in spite of the fact that they suffer a dysfunction. Partner satisfaction is also relevant, but both may have a satisfactory adjustment even though what might be considered a dysfunction exists. For instance, in the case of vaginal stenosis an older couple unable to have intercourse in the usual fashion may be satisfied when the penis is placed between the woman's legs against the clitoral area and associated with normal pelvic thrusting on the part of both partners called intrafemoral intercourse. This may spare the women discomfort and possible trauma but may bring both partners a feeling of tenderness and orgasmic satisfaction. Thus, the adjustment that a couple makes under certain circumstances may be appropriate for them although not necessarily appropriate for others.

CASE STUDY

Lila is a sixty-eight-year-old woman who underwent a mastectomy and extensive chemotherapy five years ago for a serious breast cancer. For the past five years she has been on the medication tamoxifen, and fortunately she has had no recurrence of her cancer to date. She has not been allowed to use hormone replacement therapy even vaginally because of the severity of her illness. Lila and her husband have always had a satisfactory sexual relationship, but since her therapy, her vaginal epithelium and the skin of her vulva have been very thin and crack easily when she and her husband attempt to have intercourse. Often she bleeds and is sore for several days. With time they have had intercourse less and less frequently, and because of this her vagina has narrowed and she has developed adhesions within her vagina that have made intercourse almost impossible. In spite of this, Lila and her husband have continued to kiss, caress, and fondle each other just about every night. From time to time they practice mutual masturbation, and they have, on occasion, utilized the technique of intrafemoral intercourse. Lila's husband is seventy-two years old and in good health. Both seem satisfied with their sexual adjustment, and when they were asked to describe their sexual satisfaction, they stated that it was good. Although this might be considered an unsatisfactory adjustment for many, this has allowed this couple to continue successfully with their emotional relationship.

A different couple with a similar problem has had a somewhat different adjustment.

CASE STUDY

Maureen is a fifty-year-old woman who had undergone hysterectomy and removal of both ovaries at age thirty-five because of severe endometriosis. She was then placed on hormone replacement therapy and has enjoyed good health for fifteen years. During that time she and her husband experienced excellent sexual activities and satisfaction. However, at age fifty, she was diagnosed as having a breast cancer and unfortunately had three positive lymph nodes. She was treated with a lumpectomy and radiation therapy and then was placed on tamoxifen. Shortly after recovering from her therapy, she attempted to resume intercourse and suffered a small laceration of the posterior aspect of her vaginal opening. This caused bleeding and pain and frightened her and her husband greatly. She consulted her physician, who pointed out that the vaginal epithelium and the skin of the vulva had become quite thin and that her vagina had narrowed appreciably even during the few months that therapy was instituted. Maureen became quite depressed and was placed on a mild mood elevator, which improved her outlook but not her sexual behavior. Her gynecologist prescribed 2 percent testosterone cream to be used twice a week, which helped thicken the skin of her perineum, and she was instructed to use large amounts of a water-soluble lubricant when they attempted intercourse. With patience and time, intercourse became more comfortable, and the couple was able to continue their usual sexual activities.

Fortunately, Maureen discussed this problem with her physician so that alternative therapy could be applied. Lack of estrogen often leads to thinning of the vaginal epithelium and the vulvar skin, which allows for a greater chance of vaginal and skin cracking. Tamoxifen seems to have a similar effect on these areas of the body even though it is a weak estrogen in type. For many women, testosterone cream will improve the thickness and the health of the skin and when used with a reasonable amount of lubrication can allow the couple to enjoy intercourse once again. Two lubricants designed specifically for this purpose are Replens and Astroglide. I do not personally see much difference between these, but a couple should try both to decide which one works best for them. Petroleum jelly products such as Vaseline should be avoided or only used for short periods of time, as they may have a long-term adverse effect on the skin and vaginal epithelium.

CONCLUSION

Since health care workers are often reluctant to raise issues of a sexual nature, it is reasonable for the individual woman to take control of this aspect of her life. If something is happening in your life or your relationship to interfere with sexual enjoyment, discuss it with your partner and your health care worker. Since many sexual dysfunction problems in the older woman relate to decreased sexual desire, decreased orgasmic function, or painful intercourse, these are areas that should be dealt with by a knowledgeable, caring clinical person. Relationship problems may require counseling of a different type, but directed help may be attainable after discussion with your physician or other health care worker. Many individuals suffer sexual dysfunction because of depression, which is quite common in the postmenopausal years. Often this can be alleviated with a course of antidepressant drugs or with such drugs in combination with counseling. Again, it is best to seek help rather than bear the problem. There is no reason why a healthy woman cannot enjoy sexual activity until well into old age. Maintaining this function does take effort, and it is usually effort well spent.Sexual activities do require energy and a good deal of planning and communication. Don't put it off until after the eleven o'clock news. Give it its proper place, time, and effort in your busy schedule.

CHAPTER 9

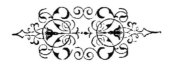

Breast Disease: Early Detection and Survival

Breast cancer is certainly a common problem in women. One out of every three new cancers in women is cancer of the breast. In 1993, there were 183,000 new cases. This is about average for the United States. Although the cumulative lifetime risk for breast cancer is that 1 in 8 women will get it, it is apparently related to age. The risk of getting breast cancer at age fifty is 2 percent, but if you live to age ninety, it will be 1 in 8.

Although the age-adjusted incidence of breast cancer has been rising, the mortality rate from this disease has been falling. According to the National Cancer Institute, there was a 30 percent increase in the incidence of breast cancer between the 1975–1979 and the 1987–1991 reporting periods among white females. The good news, however, is that the mortality rate had remained relatively flat during that time but from 1989–1992 had fallen 4.7 percent for all women. The reason for this is probably an increased awareness of breast cancer and better use of screening methods leading to earlier detection, as well as improved therapy. In spite of this improvement in survivorship, breast cancer is still the number one cancer in women and second only to lung cancer as a cause of death due to cancer in women over age fifty. Since early cancer is curable, it is important that breast cancer be detected as early as possible.

RISK FACTORS FOR BREAST CANCER

Certain factors do place women at a higher risk for breast cancer. It should be remembered, however, that most women who get breast cancer, probably in the neighborhood of 85 percent, have no significant risk factors. Therefore, screening tests are important for all women. Women at high risk are those who are in the older age category, those with a family history of breast cancer, especially in mothers or sisters, those who had started their periods at an early age, those who have never had children or who had a first full term pregnancy after the age of thirty, those who have had a history of benign breast disease, particularly requiring multiple biopsies, and those who have been found, on biopsy, to have carcinoma in situ or ductal carcinoma in situ. The term *fibrocystic disease* is not precise, and the increased fibrosis in breast disease that gives rise to this diagnosis is usually not in the tissue at risk, that is, the glandular epithelium. However, women who have had lumps and bumps in their breasts requiring biopsies more likely have hyperactivity of their glandular tissue and therefore are considered at higher risk.

Often breast cancer and ovarian cancer occur in the same family. The presence of ovarian cancer should alert the woman and physician that she may be at greater risk for developing ovarian or breast cancer in the future. Two genes indicative of high risk have been discovered on separate chromosomes and are designated the BRCA-1 gene and BRCA-2 gene. These are autosomonal dominant genes, meaning that only one gene needs to be mutated in a pair of chromosomes for the risk of cancer to be high. If such a gene is present, there is a potential of an 85 percent risk of cancer. This gene could be transmitted through the maternal and paternal lines even if the father does not have breast cancer. Although carriers of the BRCA-1 and BRCA-2 gene mutations are at high risk for developing cancer, the majority of women do not have these gene mutations. Testing, which is only done in certain centers and is quite expensive, should be reserved for those with a strong family history. Likewise, the use of prophylactic bilateral mastectomy to prevent breast cancer in such high-risk women is probably reasonable but needs to be decided upon by each woman and her physician. Such women may also decide to have their ovaries removed after completing their childbearing.

HOW IS BREAST CANCER DISCOVERED?

In order to discover breast cancer as early as possible, three important steps should be utilized by all women. The first is breast self-examination. This is something that should be performed each month, preferably just after a menstrual period. It is best accomplished with the breast wet at the time of taking a bath or shower since this allows for a sensitive appreciation of tissue change by the fingers. Performing it just after the menstrual period allows for the fact that the hormonal levels will be at their lowest and breast engorgement will be at its least, thereby allowing a true breast mass to be appreciated. In general it is difficult to appreciate a mass of much less than 0.5 cm in diameter. This is equally true for the woman and the physician. Most individuals can appreciate masses of between 0.5 and 1.0 cm if the examination is done carefully. To perform this exam it is best to be taught by a physician or health care worker the first time. The breast is a tear-shaped gland beginning in the armpit and progressing toward the midline. Therefore, the armpit should be palpated along with the area of the breast. A circular motion with the flat of the fingers should be performed starting at the edge of the breast and working toward the nipple. The breast should be thought of as a wheel, and the palpation should be performed as if it were along the spokes of a wheel. After the examination is completed, the area beneath the nipple should be palpated and the nipple should be observed for any secretions. This exercise should be performed on both breasts.

The next step in early detection is to have a breast exam by a physician at least once a year and to have the breasts examined by the physician in both the lying-down and sitting-up position. For the self-examination, it is wise to raise your arms and observe your breasts in the mirror. The examining physician should observe both breasts. Look for the symmetry of both breasts, any skin changes that may be present, and any irregularities that may be visible.

The third means of early detection is mammography. In the average woman without a significant risk factor for breast cancer, it is worthwhile to perform a baseline mammogram at about age thirty-five and then begin routine exams at age forty. Through the forties these exams may be done every one to two years. After age fifty, the American Cancer Society recommends annual examinations. Women at high risk for breast or ovarian cancer should undergo mammography beginning at the earliest age a relative has been found to have cancer, and then mammographic examinations should be repeated once a year thereafter.

WHAT DOES THE MAMMOGRAPHER LOOK FOR?

The mammographer looks for three things: new and enlarging shadows or irregular dense masses; microcalcifications in clusters or in a greater number than were seen in previous examinations; and distortions of the linear structure of the breast. Obviously masses that are developing or irregularities in the breast that are seen are reason for caution and for further evaluation. Microcalcifications are fairly common in breasts and generally do not represent cancer; however, if they are present in large numbers or increasing numbers from one exam to the next, they may represent microcalcifications in a tumor. If a density is seen it probably cannot be differentiated from a cyst of the breast. Therefore, the mammographer will usually perform an ultrasonic exam and may either work with your physician or alone to put a needle into this density to see if fluid can be removed. Cysts of the breast are very common in women before the age of menopause and in women past menopause who have had hormone replacement therapy. In general, if clear or yellowish fluid is removed and the mass disappears, it is probably a benign cyst and need not be evaluated further. On the other hand, if the mass does not disappear with removal of fluid or the fluid is greenish or bloody, a biopsy is indicated.

If a mammographer sees an increasing number of microcalcifications in a cluster, a biopsy should be performed. Also, local breast thickening or visible change from previous exams should be biopsied. Some rapidly developing tumors can cause pain and tenderness, but in most cases early breast cancer is painless. Spontaneous nipple discharge, particularly in one breast only, is worthy of further evaluation but may be present in several benign conditions.

It should be noted that even when enough abnormalities are present in a mammographic exam to warrant a biopsy, only about 25 percent of patients will actually have breast cancer. Therefore, if your physician calls to say you require a biopsy, don't panic. You still have a 3 out of 4 chance of this being a benign condition. Also, it is important to pick up breast tumors as early as possible so that they may be dealt with before they metastasize to other parts of the body. In general, breast cancer first goes to lymph nodes but then may go to distant sites such as lung and bone. The smaller the tumor, the less likely this is to happen, and the more likely the chances are that the patient will be cured. Most breast cancers grow very slowly, doubling in size about every year. Therefore, a breast cancer that is 1 cm in diameter has probably been present for about six to eight years. This is why early detection is more likely to catch the tumor before it has a chance to spread.

A very strong rule in medicine today is not to sit and watch a lump get larger. If you have a lump, report it to your physician. Your physician may order a mammogram simply to see if the lump could be a cyst. Your physician may also put a needle into the mass on your first visit to see if it is filled with fluid. Masses that persist should be biopsied regardless of whether or not the mammogram suggests an abnormality.

A few tumors are very aggressive and grow very rapidly. Although these will generally require a great deal more therapy than just removing the mass, they are no longer the hopeless situations they once were. We now have excellent chemotherapy as well as surgical and radiologic techniques for treatment. Cures are possible, but it is important that a physician be consulted as early as possible.

BIOPSING THE BREAST

There are several ways to biopsy the breast. The first is fine needle aspiration. Usually this is carried out under ultrasound guidance or, if the mass is large enough, as an office procedure without ultrasound. This will give both fluid and tissue for pathologic evaluation. In many studies the agreement between such biopsies and the findings in masses after removal is 100 percent for determining whether a cancer is present. Fine needle biopsies can be performed in the office in about twenty to thirty minutes. Often the radiologist will perform this if an ultrasound reveals a cystic mass.

Open biopsies are often performed in a surgicenter under local anesthesia. This can be carried out relatively easily if there is a palpable mass. However, if an area of microcalcification is noted on the mammogram but no mass is palpable, the biopsy can be carried out using a stereotactic needle technique. In the past, wires were inserted into the breast, under X-ray guidance, so that open biopsy could be performed using the wire as the guide. With stereotactic needle technique, fine needle aspiration of several areas involving the microcalcification region can be carried out. While this technique has not replaced open surgical biopsy, it is very useful for small lesions seen only on mammography.

To summarize, it is extremely important that women utilize breast self-examination, routine examination by a physician, and mammography to detect breast tumors as early as possible. Suspicious areas should be further examined by fine needle aspiration or biopsies. Lumps or masses should never be ignored until a specific diagnosis is made. Although mammography has been stated to be less accurate in younger women because of the greater density of their breasts, it should still be used because it is superior to no evaluation at all. A cancer that is detected in a younger woman may be curable. If it is ignored because routine evaluation has not taken place, it will most likely be lethal in the long run.

STAGING AND TREATMENT

When a diagnosis of breast cancer is made by biopsy, it is important to stage the cancer so that the appropriate therapy may be selected. This is done by inspecting the histology of the tumor, measuring the size of the tumor, and evaluating the lymph nodes that drain the breast. In addition, the patient should have a chest X ray or CT scan and liver function studies to be sure that the tumor has not spread to the chest or liver. The physician will probably also order a bone scan even though it is likely to be positive in only 2 to 3 percent of women with tumors under 2 cm. Most physicians advise a baseline bone scan in patients who have breast cancer and who will be followed for a long period of time.

Clinical Stage I are tumors of up to 2 cm in diameter. Clinical Stage II are tumors that are 2 to 5 cm in diameter. Clinical Stage III are tumors larger than 5 cm or those that have skin involvement or are more histologically aggressive cancers. Pathologists will also evaluate the cancers for the presence of estrogen and progesterone receptor proteins. Not only is this information helpful in designing therapy, but it has prognostic implications as well. It may also help the oncologist to decide which chemotherapy should be offered.

For individuals with invasive breast cancer of Stage I or II, studies have shown that lumpectomy plus irradiation is as likely to be successful as is mastectomy. On the other hand, positive lymph nodes can be treated with appropriate chemotherapy whether mastectomy or breast preservation is utilized. If there is more than one cancer within the same breast or if the breast will be grossly deformed by removal of the mass, a mastectomy is probably a better course to follow. Modern surgeons design the operation so that breast reconstruction is possible should the patient desire this. In Stage I and II breast cancers, chest muscles can be spared and normal function can be maintained. If a node dissection and irradiation have been carried out, there is some chance of swelling of the arm, and the patient may be required to wear an elastic support on the arm, at least for a period of time.

For women with disease that has metastasized to lymph nodes or distant sites, the physician will probably prescribe adjunctive chemotherapy. Currently, newer techniques utilizing chemotherapeutic agents such as Adriamycin, Cisplatin, and other platinum-containing medications and Taxol have been very useful in prolonging life or helping to effect cures. The weak estrogen tamoxifen has been used prophylactically in women with early metastatic disease and is currently being used for about five years after original treatment of the tumor. It is beyond the scope of this book to discuss therapeutic regimens with chemotherapy or tamoxifen, as each woman with breast cancer should be treated individually with therapy designed by a competent oncologist.

CONCLUSION

It is vital for every woman to learn breast self-examination early and to continue it throughout life; to see her physician regularly for a breast examination; and to use mammography according to the American Cancer Society guidelines (see Table 9.1). If you get a telephone call from your physician suggesting further mammographic

TABLE 9.1.   American Cancer Society Guidelines
for Mammography

Baseline mammography for all women	age 35–40
Mammography every 1–2 years	age 40–49
Annual mammography	after age 50

views, don't panic. This is a common phenomenon, and additional pictures will usually clear up an unclear situation without the need for further testing or therapy. If
your physician suggests an ultrasound exam and a fine needle aspiration, again
remember that the majority of women who undergo these procedures still do not have
cancer. If you have a lump, work with your physician to resolve whether or not it is a
serious problem. Do not put it off. Finally, if a diagnosis of cancer is made, do not
panic. The majority of women still get cured, particularly if it is an early lesion, and
the therapies available today are improved over what we had to work with in the past.
The important thing is to use the detection methods to make an early diagnosis so that
treatment may be kept to a minimum and cure rates kept at their highest level.

CHAPTER 10

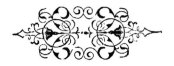

High Blood Pressure, Heart Disease, and Stroke

Hypertension is a common condition, but rarely does it have associated symptoms. It occurs equally in men and women. The National Health Survey carried out between 1976 and 1980 determined that 44 percent of whites and 60 percent of African Americans between the ages of sixty-five and seventy-four were hypertensive. This diagnosis was made on the basis of three consecutive blood pressure readings taken on a single visit that were greater than 160/95. At that time, the World Health Organization also recognized 160/95 as the beginning level of hypertension, but since that time studies have shown that even lower blood pressures are associated with higher than average incidences of myocardial infarction, stroke, and death. Recently, the fifth report of the Joint National Committee for Detection, Evaluation, and Treatment of High Blood Pressure set the level at 130/85 as the high of normal. Blood pressure does rise gradually with age, and often elderly people will demonstrate elevated systolic levels of blood pressure without necessarily elevating their diastolic pressure. Because this probably reflects an increase in the stiffness of the walls of the arteries that occurs gradually with age, it has been suggested that hypertension in the elderly occurs when the blood pressure is greater than 140/90.

The fifth report of the Joint National Committee, which was published in 1993, classified hypertension into normal, high normal, and hypertensive levels for people eighteen years and older. Table 10.1 outlines this classification.

Discovering hypertension is important so that lifestyle changes and possibly treatment can take place early. The Systolic Hypertension in the Elderly Program (SHEP) reported in 1991 that there were 36 percent fewer fatal than nonfatal strokes and 27 percent fewer fatal than nonfatal myocardial infarctions in actively treated elderly persons as compared with placebo control groups. These benefits were noted across all age, race, gender, and blood pressure subgroups. There did not seem to be an advantage in one treatment method over another.

The diagnosis of hypertension is not always easy. It is important to take the blood

TABLE 10.1.   Classification of Blood Pressure for Adults Ages 18 and Older

	Systolic mm of mercury	Diastolic mm of mercury
Normal	Less than 130	Less than 85
High normal	130–139	85–89
Hypertension		
Mild	140–159	90–99
Moderate	160–179	100–109
Severe	180–209	110–119
Very severe	Greater than 210	Greater than 120

pressure after at least five minutes of rest, to use a blood pressure cuff that covers about 80 percent of the upper arm to position at about the level of the heart, and to repeat the blood pressure at least three times if it is elevated. A variety of stresses, including going to the doctor, make the blood pressure appear elevated. Even if the blood pressure is elevated in the physician's office, it should be repeated several times under more relaxed and normal conditions. Fire stations and pharmacies often offer blood pressure checks, and someone who is considered to be a potential hypertensive should purchase a blood pressure cuff and have a friend or family member learn to take her blood pressure. It is then possible to repeat the blood pressure studies when she is relaxed. Since blood pressure elevation occurs in 15 to 20 percent of the adult population, and since it does relate to the risk of death due to coronary artery disease, stroke, and damage to other organs such as the eyes and the kidneys, it is important from a public health standpoint as well as from the standpoint of a woman's own health to detect this condition early and, if necessary, treat it.

TREATMENT OF HYPERTENSION

If normal or high normal blood pressure in the older woman is 140/90 or less, she does not need specific therapy. Since smoking is a risk factor for hypertension, certainly this is another reason to encourage her to stop smoking. There has been a great deal of discussion about proper diet in both the treatment and prevention of hypertension. The majority of the controversy is centered about the issue of salt in the diet. There is some recent evidence that a normotensive person does not need to reduce the amount of salt in the diet, but this has come from population studies and probably does not take into consideration the fact that some individuals are more salt sensitive. It is difficult to know whether someone who is salt sensitive and normotensive will become hypertensive if she is kept on a diet with normal amounts of salt, or whether she will be protected from developing hypertension later if she does reduce the amount of salt in her diet. Nevertheless, it is probably reasonable to limit salt intake to a moderate level, which is 1.5 to 2.5 grams of sodium per day. It is best for hypertensive people to reduce the amount of salt below this level, or as low as they can tolerate. For women wishing to find a diet that will help prevent hypertension, and for those who are already hypertensive, dietary changes that may contribute to lowering the blood pressure are those that increase the amount of calcium, magnesium, and potassium in the diet. Moderating the use of alcohol, increasing fiber, and decreasing saturated fat is also important. Weight loss to as close to lean body mass as possible is very helpful in treating hypertension, and exercise particularly of the endurance-developing type, such as brisk walking, swimming, or aerobics, is very helpful. Individuals classified as mild hypertensives, that is, those with a systolic blood pressure of 140 to 159 and diastolic blood pressures of 90 to 99, often will reduce their blood pressures 10 to 20 mm of mercury in this way without requiring further treatment. Diet change, weight reduction, and exercise are a part of the treatment of all hypertensives, and this may be all that is necessary for the milder types of hypertension.

For those who do not respond to diet and exercise or who are already classified as moderate to severe hypertensives, drug therapy is probably indicated. This should certainly be undertaken under the careful control of a physician. In general, therapy is begun with the lowest possible dose of a drug, increasing it only to obtain the desired response in an individual patient. Overtreatment can be quite dangerous, and an abrupt lowering of the blood pressure may cause fainting and, in those who already have coronary artery disease, may decrease the profusion of the coronary arteries, leading to symptoms of heart attack. It is also important to keep the dose of antihypertensive drugs as low as possible, because they do cause many side effects. Often they reduce the amount of calcium in the bloodstream, which can lead to a slowing of the heart rate or arrhythmias. In addition, they often cause an elevation of LDL cholesterol (plasma low density lipoprotein) and HDL cholesterol (plasma high density lipoproteins). They also often reduce kidney and liver function. People taking antihypertensive drugs, particularly in higher doses, often complain of tiredness and weakness, and some may develop depression. Several of the antihypertensive drugs decrease libido in the male and may cause impotence. The treatment of hypertension is a serious matter that requires the cooperation and careful attention to the needs of the patient by both the patient and her physician.

A variety of types of antihypertension drugs are available. These include diuretics such as hydrocholorathiazide, or other agents containing hydrocholorathiazide, and a variety of other diuretics that have been developed to act on different areas of the kidney. Many of these spare potassium, preventing the side effects of low potassium. The beta blockers such as propranolol, Atenolol, Carteolol, and other agents that block both the alpha- and beta-receptors of the blood vessel walls act directly on them to cause dilation. They are all very effective in reducing blood pressure but may have a variety of side effects. Calcium channel blockers (calcium antagonists) are effective in reducing blood pressure, but they sometimes cause difficulty with heart function, for example, conduction defects.

One group of medications, the angiotensin-converting enzyme inhibitors (ACEs), are now very popular and effective. Perhaps one of the best known of these is Vasotec, which is one of the most often prescribed medications in the United States today. Studies have found no particularly significant differences in the effects on quality of life in women and men using any of these agents. At the present time, there is not sufficient data to determine which may be better for women versus men. Unfortunately, many of the studies done to this point have been done only on men. All these medications, however, seem to be effective in the treatment of women with hypertension.

The objective of treatment should be to reduce the blood pressure to 140/90 or somewhat below this level. Studies have shown that when blood pressures are higher than 140/90 in older people, there is a marked increase in cardiovascular disease. Hypertension may be detected and managed as a patient is seen for her routine health care visits.

CASE STUDY

Ellie is a 55-year-old divorced woman working as an accountant in city government. She has two grown children and has always been in good health. She went through menopause at age fifty-one and is on hormone replacement therapy consisting of daily estrogen and progesterone. When seen for her annual health maintenance visit, she was noted to be in general good health, but her blood pressure, on the day she was seen, was 160/90. Ellie is five feet, four inches tall, and a year before she had a blood pressure of 130/80 and a weight of 150 pounds. Her weight was 160 pounds. She stated that she had been working extremely hard, often twelve-hour days, and she has been under some stress from a male supervisor who she felt would like to eliminate her job. She stated that other older women in the office had recently either resigned or transferred to other offices. When asked about exercise, she stated that she does not have time. When asked about sleep, she stated that she will frequently fall asleep easily because she is very tired but will awaken at 2:00 or 3:00 A.M. and then be unable to go back to sleep. Routine laboratory studies obtained at the visit were completely normal except for a somewhat elevated cholesterol of 225. Her LDL cholesterol was slightly elevated, and her HDL cholesterol was on the low side of normal at 40.

We discussed at length her diet and the need for exercise, and she agreed that she would go on a low-fat, low-cholesterol diet, take walks in the evening, and use her exercycle. She stated that she could have blood pressures taken at her pharmacy, and we arranged for her to have this done, preferably on weekends when the stress of her job would not be great. We planned to meet in two months.

When she returned, she had lost 6 pounds and stated that she was sleeping better, although she was still waking up early in the morning. The pressures at work had not changed much, but she was making a strong effort to leave her concerns at work and find other things to occupy her mind in the evening. She stated that she had joined the YWCA and had enrolled in an aerobic exercise class, which she attended three evenings a week. She had met some other women in similar circumstances, and they had begun to do some social activities together.

(continued)

CASE STUDY (CONTINUED)

Blood pressures taken at her pharmacy on the weekends had been consistently below 140/90. She stated that she felt much better about the way things were going and would return only before the date of her health maintenance visit if she noted changes in her blood pressure.

About eight months later, she returned because her blood pressure at the pharmacy had been 150/90. Because her blood pressure had continued to be below 140/90, she had not had it checked for about five months. Although she had continued exercising a few times each week and had been able to stay on her diet, she had not lost any more weight. Her problems at work had remained about the same, but she stated that she was still sleeping better, and was surprised to find that her blood pressure was elevated. In the office, her blood pressure was 160/90. Her total cholesterol, on this visit was 210.

Because I felt that she was following her diet to a certain extent and getting exercise, but was still in a stressful occupation, and because her blood pressure elevation seemed to be progressing, I referred her to an internist. The internist advised antihypertensive drug therapy. The results of the consultation did not yield any new medical facts or discover new physical disabilities, but the internist did feel it was reasonable to start medication. Ellie was prescribed a diuretic, which brought her blood pressure once again below 140/90, where it has stayed for the past two years.

This is a very typical history of a woman who is somewhat overweight, leading a stressful life, probably not getting as much exercise as would be healthy, and who has developed essential hypertension over time. In the early stages, it was entirely reasonable to attempt to treat her with diet, exercise, and, where possible, decreasing stress. However, as her condition progressed, medical therapy became necessary. The important thing to remember is that hypertension is not a static illness and therefore must be monitored to be sure it does not progress. If it does, therapy should be instituted so that it does not contribute to other cardiovascular diseases.

CARDIOVASCULAR DISEASE

The most common cardiovascular disease is coronary artery disease. This is a condition in which the arteries to the heart are narrowed or blocked by atherosclerotic plaques in their walls. When this occurs the blood supply to the heart muscles is reduced and may lead to angina (chest pain) or a heart attack (myocardial infarction). Fortunately, screening is very effective and therefore knowing the risk factors and trying to eliminate as many of these as possible should reduce the risk for the individual woman. The risk factors are listed in Table 10.2. Certainly, she should be encouraged to stop smoking. Hypertension should be detected and treated, and diabetes should also be detected and controlled. Women who are past the age of fifty-five or who have

TABLE 10.2.   Risk Factor for Coronary Artery Disease

Cigarette smoking

Hypertension

Diabetes mellitis

Age over 55 (for women)

Early menopause without hormone replacement

Family history of premature coronary artery disease

HDL less than 35 mg/dl

Obesity

Physical inactivity

undergone a premature menopause should be on estrogen replacement therapy, if there is no contraindication, as estrogen has a positive effect on cholesterol, lowering total cholesterol and LDL and elevating HDL. Estrogen also acts an antioxidant, helps to remove ateriosclerotic plaques from the coronary arteries, and also seems to cause dilation of the coronary arteries. For people with a family history of premature coronary disease, every effort should be made to control cholesterol. For those who are found to have a low HDL (below 35 mg per dl), an exercise program that is important for everyone should certainly be advised. Diet should be controlled and obesity treated. With these steps, it should be possible to help many women avoid coronary artery disease and its serious consequences.

Again, with coronary artery disease, most studies have been done in men. It is not always possible to apply these findings to women. One of the striking differences between the sexes is the implication of chest pain (angina). In a large study in Framingham, Massachusetts, it was suggested that coronary artery disease in women had a more favorable outcome than in men and that angina observed in the females in the study rarely progressed to myocardial infarction. Angina occurred in 56 percent of the women in this study as compared to 43 percent in the men. Only 14 percent of the women with angina progressed to myocardial infarction within five years, as compared to 25 percent of the men. However, when angiograms were used to study coronary arteries, it turned out that a large proportion of women suffering from angina really had noncardiac chest pain. In the early 1980s, the Coronary Artery Surgery Study (CASS) noted that when angiograms were applied, 50 percent of women with angina were found to have normal coronary arteries. Only 17 percent of men with angina had normal coronary arteries. The Framingham Study, which did a follow-up study of its subjects for twenty-six years, noted that 40 percent of coronary artery disease occurred in women. Older women with angina had the same adverse outcome as did men. This is a similar finding to one reported by the Cleveland Clinic, which found that 90 percent of postmenopausal women with suspect angina who underwent angiography had significant coronary artery disease, compared to fifty percent of premenopausal women. It seems that chest pain in younger women may be due to a variety of reasons, whereas chest pain in older women is frequently caused by coronary artery disease and should be taken seriously.

The risk of coronary artery disease in women is lower than it is in men until about age sixty to sixty-five, at which time it becomes equal to men and goes up rapidly, as does the risk in men. Each year, 2 1/2 million women are hospitalized in the United States because of cardiovascular disease, and of these five hundred thousand will die, with half the deaths being attributed to coronary artery disease. These are many more women than will die of cancer or other causes.

STROKE

Cerebral vascular disease, or stroke, is the second most common cardiovascular disease after coronary artery disease and is the third leading cause of death in the United States, exceeded only by heart disease and cancer. Risk factors for stroke are high blood pressure, smoking, and diabetes. Therefore, smoking cessation and the treatment of hypertension and diabetes help to decrease the incidence of stroke in women. If coronary artery disease is present, this also is a risk factor for stroke.Stroke is a vascular accident in the brain. It may be a hemorrhage or it may be a thrombosis, the coagulation of blood within a vessel. Both can be lethal or can cause neurological impairment or paralysis. In older people, if death does not take place, multiple infarcts in the brain may lead to dementia. Certainly this is a condition of serious consequence that should be avoided if possible. Stroke prevention is another area in which estrogen replacement seems to be of value. In the National Health and Nutrition Exam Survey carried out between 1971 and 1987, it was noted that the incidence of stroke per 10,000 was 124 if no hormone replacement therapy was being used and only 82 if it was. This translated into a reduction in risk of about 30 percent and led to the conclusion that estrogen had a cerebral vascular protective effect. Many women worry about thrombosis occurring with estrogen use because of the increased incidence of thrombosis that has been reported to be associated in the past with birth control pills, particularly with high-dose birth control pills. It should be noted that the estrogen in estrogen replacement therapy has only one fifth the potency of the estrogen in even the lowest dose of contraceptives. This dose has been shown to have no effect on systolic or diastolic blood pressure. In the vast majority of women, it does not cause thrombosis. Furthermore, women with hypertension, coronary artery disease, or a history of stroke can take estrogen. While birth control pills have, at times, been reported to affect systolic blood pressure in some women, estrogen replacement therapy usually does not. The evidence indicates that the majority of women who are hypertensive and on medication can safely take estrogen.

CONCLUSION

There is no question that hypertension, with its associated coronary artery disease and stroke, certainly accounts for a large percentage of deaths in women, particularly in the elderly. It is a much greater hazard for death and disability than is cancer. The best therapy is prevention, which implies such commonsense practices as stopping smoking, using alcohol in moderation, following a good diet, maintaining weight within normal limits, getting moderate exercise, and being tested regularly, usually at annual health visits, for hypertension. Attention to cholesterol control is important, as elevated cholesterol and LDL is a risk factor for coronary heart disease. All of these activities are within the woman's own control. Certainly, if hypertension or coronary artery disease is diagnosed or the woman is unfortunate enough to have a stroke, there are good medications available to help prevent future problems. Used properly with the help of a physician, they can increase life expectancy.

CHAPTER 11

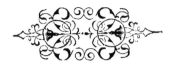

The Cancer Risk

Cancer is the second leading cause of death in older women. It is, however, only half as common as death due to heart disease. In women over the age of sixty-five, deaths due to heart disease occur at a rate of 1,735 per 100,000 women, and cancer deaths are 871 per 100,000. The number of deaths due to cancer is twice the number of deaths due to stroke (423 per 100,000). Since women live longer some cancers are either in places where they can be detected early or give symptoms early enough to allow a good cure rate. Cancers of the skin, cervix, uterus, breast, and vulva are examples of these. Other cancers are relatively "silent" and do not cause symptoms until they are quite far advanced. Cancers of the ovaries, lungs, and pancreas fall into this category. In general, the earlier a cancer can be detected, the more likelihood there is for a cure and the more likely it will be that the cancer and its treatment will cause fewer death. Where screening programs are available for cancers that are frequently seen in women, they should be utilized.

Table 11.1 depicts the 1990 cancer death rates (deaths per 100,000 population) in females age sixty-five and over. For all groups, 65–74, 75–84, and 85 and over, the death rate due to lung cancer is high, probably relating to the smoking history of women in that particular age group. From age seventy-five on, the highest death rate from cancer is in cancers of the digestive tract. Breast cancer, which is perhaps feared the most by women because it is the most common, ranks third in all three age groups as far as death rate is concerned. It does increase with each decade, because the incidence of breast cancer increases with age. Likewise, genital cancers, which represent the fourth category of risk in older women, increase with each decade, while cancers of the lymphatic system (lymphomas), urinary system, and leukemia remain the next most common causes of death due to cancer in this age group.

TABLE 11.1.   Cancer Death Rates (per 100,000 Population) in Females Aged 65 and Over (1980)

Age Group	Type of Cancer	Death Rate
65–74	Lung	181.7
	Digestive organs	153.0
	Breast	111.7
	Genital organs	71.0
	Lymphatic tissue and blood	39.5
	Urinary	19.8
	Leukemia	18.8
75–84	Lung	194.5
	Digestive organs	293.3
	Breast	146.3
	Genital organs	95.3
	Lymphatic tissue and blood	71.2
	Urinary	38.5
	Leukemia	38.8
85 and over	Lung	142.8
	Digestive organs	497.6
	Breast	196.8
	Genital organs	115.6
	Lymphatic tissue and blood	90.0
	Urinary	68.5
	Leukemia	65.0

LUNG CANCER

The incidence of lung cancer increases steadily throughout a woman's life. Survival rates decrease with increasing age. Screening programs using routine chest X rays or the evaluation of sputum for cancer cells have not proven to be cost effective for the general population. But these programs have not been studied in older women alone, among whom the incidence is higher. Generally, screening programs do best in populations in which the incidence of a disease is high, and the test is useful for picking up early lesions. It may be that chest X ray or sputum analysis may have a place in screening for early disease in older women, but currently no such programs are in effect or being tried. My feeling has always been that smokers, particularly those who have smoked heavily for long periods of time, should be followed with routine chest X rays every few years. That is my personal opinion, and other physicians may not agree. Whether or not screening is applied, prevention is still important, which means stopping smoking. The incidence of lung cancer has gone up in women and down in men, primarily because fewer men are now smoking but more women have taken up the habit. Stopping smoking will not be entirely protective, but it will decrease the risk of lung cancer by as much as 80 percent over time.

The earliest symptom of lung cancer is cough. Bloody sputum is less common (about 20 percent) and usually indicative of a lesion in one of the larger bronchi. At times, pneumonia occurs because a portion of the lung is blocked by the cancer. In advanced disease, the patient may complain of pain in the shoulder or arm, may develop edema of the upper body because of a block of the return of blood through the upper chest to the heart, and may experience hoarseness, shortness of breath, and air hunger. The size of the lesion can usually be delineated with a CT (computed tomography) scan and the diagnosis made specifically by fine needle aspiration or by bronchoscopy (the placement of a tube through the trachea and into a bronchus of the lung to obtain washings or biopsy). The exact means for making a specific diagnosis depends upon the size and location of the lesion. At times, the lymph nodes above the clavicle (collar bone) may be enlarged, and biopsying these may provide the diagnosis.

There are several different cell types that cause lung cancer, and the treatment depends upon how far the tumor has spread and the type of cancer that it may be. The most common lung cancer in women is adenocarcinoma. If the lesion is early, removing part of the lung (lobectomy) is indicated. At times, if the tumor in the lung is large and not operable, it may decrease in size with chemotherapy and irradiation or a combination thereof, and then be resectable. The protocols for the use of chemotherapy in certain types of lung cancer and the overall prognosis depend upon the type of cell involved in the cancer and the size of the tumor as well as its metastatic spread. Again, it is better to avoid the disease than to have to treat it. Every year there are seventy thousand new cases of lung cancer in American women, with the death rate overall of 23 per 100,000. In smokers the risk of lung cancer is increased 730 fold. Smoking has an attributable risk to the development of lung cancer of 87 percent. That means that when all risk factors are considered, smoking is overwhelmingly the largest reason for developing lung cancer. It is important that you don't smoke, and if you do smoke, stop immediately.

BREAST CANCER

Breast cancer is the most common cancer in American women, with 182,000 new cases per year. The death rate is 22 per 100,000, making it less than the death rate for lung cancer. The reason for this is that breast cancer can often be detected in earlier stages and can be cured. Also, there is quite good therapy and many patients can be salvaged. Breast cancer risk increases with age, by the age of sixty-five, the risk is 1 in 17, and by age eighty-five, the risk is 1 in 9. In fact, age is the most significant risk factor for cancer of the breast. Therefore, surveillance should go on throughout the woman's life. It is a sad commentary that a recent study showed that fewer than forty percent of physicians routinely screen patients over the age of sixty-five, and only 21 percent routinely screen women over the age of seventy-five. While breast self-examination and examination annually by a physician are strongly recommend, mammography is still a major screening tool. The American Cancer Society recommends yearly mammography after age fifty and strongly encourages women to continue breast self-examination.

Other risk factors beside age are a history of having had a previous breast cancer, a first-degree relative (a mother or a sister) with breast cancer, early age of onset of menses (usually before age twelve), late first full-term pregnancy (usually after age thirty), and prior irradiation to the chest for other reasons. I reiterate the following reminders:

1. Get an annual mammogram.
2. Continue to do breast self-examination, and have your breasts examined by a physician at least once a year.
3. If a lump is found, it needs to be evaluated, even if the mammogram is negative.

COLORECTAL CANCER

The third most common cause of cancer deaths in women is colorectal cancer, which affects older women more commonly than younger women with the majority of cases occurring after age sixty-five. The maximum incidence of disease is at age eighty.

Risk factors for colorectal cancer include a long-term use of high-fat, high-calorie diets, a history of polyps of the colon, previous colon cancer, or inflammatory bowel disease such as ulcerative colitis. People in families in which the disease has been prevalent should be screened even if they are asymptomatic. Many physicians feel that prevention can be aided by eating diets high in calcium, vitamin C, and vitamin D, which act by blocking promoters of neoplastic growth. A diet high in fiber is also recommended.

There are several ways of screening for bowel and rectal cancer. The easiest and least expensive is to screen stool at least on three occasions annually for the presence of occult blood. Small hemacult cards are available on which the stool samples may be spread. The cards may then be taken to the physician's office, where they can be developed for signs of occult blood. Unfortunately, several tumors are missed using this method only because it relies on the fact that the tumor is shedding blood, at least in small amounts. Because several foods, such as horseradish and cauliflower, contain substances that may give a false positive test, so the presence of apparent occult blood does not prove that there is a lesion, and the absence does not prove that there is not. Certainly, any evidence for rectal bleeding, even if the patient has hemorrhoids, should be investigated. The means of investigating this are sigmoidoscopy or colonoscopy. Sigmoidoscopy allows investigation of the lower bowel. Since about 80 percent of lesions are in this region, it is quite good at detecting colon cancer. However, if sigmoidoscopy is negative and the patient has been experiencing rectal bleeding, if there is a strong family history of colorectal cancer or polyps, or if there is a history of previous polyps in the patient, a colonoscopy should be performed. This allows visualization of the entire colon. The American Cancer Society suggests that a rectal examination, which will pick up cancer of the rectum and lower colon in many patients, and a fecal occult blood test be performed annually on everyone over the age of fifty. Sigmoidoscopy should then be performed every three to five years. Colonoscopy can be utilized for people who bleed, for those with strong family histories of colorectal cancer, or for those who have had previous polyps. In general, many gastroenterologists feel that the majority of bowel cancers develop in colon polyps of the adenomatous type and that it may take up to ten years for such polyps to develop into cancers. Although there is some discussion as to whether or not colonoscopy needs to be performed more frequently than every ten years, it is likely that these guidelines will change from time to time. Certainly people who have rectal bleeding or those with strong risk factors for colorectal cancer should be screened aggressively.

Aside from rectal bleeding, changes in bowel habits should lead to an investigation for colon cancer. These changes may include diarrhea or diarrhea intermittent with constipation. The presence of painful bowel movement, urgency to move the bowel, crampiness, and weight loss are usually more advanced symptoms. In very advanced cases, obstruction of the colon or perforation may actually take place.

For the best prognosis, it is desirable that the disease be found in its local stage, but the disease is often found in a more advanced stage in women past the age of sixty-five. Women of advancing age have a lower survival rate than do younger women, but the reason for this is not known.

Treatment for colorectal disease is primarily surgical, allowing for a wide excision of the region of the bowel that contains the cancer. If positive lymph nodes or further spread are noted, the likelihood is a poor prognosis. There are several chemotherapy protocols being evaluated for colon cancer at the present time that may increase survival in patients with rectal and anal cancers.

Again, screening for this disease to make an early diagnosis is the most important thing that can be done to prevent the high mortality rate in this disease. If you note rectal bleeding or changes in your bowel habits or other GI symptoms, this should be reported to your physician and an evaluation begun. If your history indicates a high risk for this disease, a routine surveillance should be instituted. If you have been treated for colorectal cancer, frequent follow-up with physical examination and colonoscopy for the rest of your life is indicated.

CASE STUDY

Joan who is sixty-eight years old and a widow, came to me for the first time for a health maintenance visit. She has had no physical complaints, and her physical examination was completely within normal limits. However, she did state that her father died of colon cancer and that two of her brothers had polyps removed from their colons. She had never had a screening study of any kind. Her bowel function was normal, and she was given hemacult tests annually by her family physician. She exercises regularly, eats a healthy diet, and felt that her risk of cancer was probably low. During her physical examination, a rectal exam was performed and was negative. Some stool was present in the rectum and was applied to a hemacult card, which proved to be negative for occult blood. Because of her family history and the fact that she had never been screened, I suggested a sigmoidoscopy and referred her to our gastroenterologist for this purpose. The gastroenterologist decided to perform a complete colonoscopy and found an adenomatous polyp high in her colon, beyond what would have been seen by sigmoidoscopy. The patient had been given a good bowel cleaning prior to her colonoscopy, and the gastroenterologist was able to remove the polyp through the colonoscope. No other polyps or lesions were seen. The pathology report cited an area of adenocarcinoma present at the tip of the polyp. The base of the polyp was negative for tumor, and the gastroenterologist felt that this was all the therapy that Joan needed. It is planned to rescreen Joan with a colonoscopy in one year. If this is negative, she will then be screened every two to three years.

This is the best possible outcome, and it demonstrates that early cancers do develop in polyps in many patients. The fact that Joan had a positive family history for both polyps and colon cancer was a risk factor necessitating that she be tested with colonoscopy at reasonable intervals, making it possible to detect the disease early and with minimal therapy required. She will require continuous follow-up for the rest of her life.

CANCERS OF THE REPRODUCTIVE ORGANS

Cancers of the reproductive organs are the fourth most common reason for cancer deaths in older women as a group. However, they are all different cancers, and some can be detected early because of the likelihood of being seen on physical examination (vulvar and vaginal cancers), because of screening tests such as the Pap smear (cervical cancer), or because of a high likelihood of bleeding in early lesions (endometrial cancer). On the other hand, ovarian and tubal cancers are silent cancers until they progress to a fairly advanced stage. The majority of advanced genital cancers are cancers of the ovary. Fortunately, tubal cancer is rare and does not contribute a great deal to the number of cancer deaths.

Vulvar Cancer

Cancer of the vulva is actually a skin cancer. Most of the cell types are squamous cell, which are derived from the cells that cover the skin. In many cases, squamous cells evolve through various cell changes in the skin that are benign at first, and then may be malignant but superficial (carcinoma in situ). Each of the lesions are relatively easy to treat and control and are completely curable. When the cancer does develop and invade, the treatment necessarily becomes more involved. The larger the tumor and the deeper the invasion, the poorer the prognosis. This is a tumor that can be detected early, even in its precancerous form, by paying attention to skin changes in the vulva. With early detection, good outcomes can be anticipated. Unfortunately, diagnosis and therapy is often delayed because of both patient and physician neglect. Older women do not examine their vulvar regions often, and if skin changes in the form of pimples, bumps, or lumps develop, they are often ignored until they become quite large or cause pain or itching. When itching or pain occurs, which is fairly frequent in such lesions, they may be treated with creams and salves purchased at the drugstore, again for a relatively long period of time. Also, physicians who are not used to dealing with vulvar lesions may prescribe a variety of local medications rather than perform a biopsy. The bottom line is that all new lesions of the skin should be biopsed, as should skin that is chronically itchy, burning, or uncomfortable.

Actually, 50 percent of vulvar cancers arise from skin changes classified as vulvar dystrophies. There are a variety of these, but each has malignant potential. At times, the skin in the area becomes very thin and loses its pigmentation and hair follicles, causing itching and burning. If a woman is sexually active, there may be cracking associated with sexual intercourse (lichen sclerosis et atrophicus). When such a condition arises, biopsies should be performed to rule out carcinoma. Other types of dystrophies of the hypertrophic variety involve a thickening and piling up of the cells of the skin and often a raised or darkened lesion. This too should be biopsied. Fortunately, the overall incidence of invasive carcinoma in the vulvar dystrophies is low, about 2 to 4 percent. Early diagnosis depends upon biopsy.

Skin biopsy can be carried out using a small disposable punch instrument. All that is required is that a small amount of local anesthesia, such as xylocaine, be injected into the skin, followed by the application of a skin punch that will yield a small piece of skin for tissue evaluation. Usually, all that is required to control bleeding is chemical cautery with silver nitrate. Occasionally, a stitch needs to be taken. Generally the area of dystrophy is fairly extensive, and multiple biopsies may be necessary.

Treatment of the dystrophies is necessary to prevent the development of cancer. Once a cancer is diagnosed, the therapy and prognosis depend upon the extent of the tumor. Tumors that have not invaded the basal membrane of the skin, that is, those that are designated as carcinoma in situ, may be managed with a generous local excision. If the tumor is arising in an area of dystrophy, it is important that the entire area of dystrophy be treated. Minimally invasive tumors, those that have not gone beyond 1 to 2 mm below the skin basement membrane, can also be treated by wide excision. Larger tumors and the tumors that have invaded can be managed by wide excision, by partial vulvectomy, or by radial vulvectomy, depending upon their extent. Lymph node dissection of the groin nodes on the same side as the tumor for smaller tumors and on both sides for larger ones is also performed. If lymph nodes are positive for tumor in the groin, irradiation therapy is usually applied as well, to destroy tumors in the deeper nodal areas.

Recently, many cancer treatment centers have begun to use a technique called Mohs surgery, which was developed by a dermatologist and limits the extent of the removal of the tumor by removing small amounts of skin beyond the obvious margin of the tumor and immediately subjecting them to histologic evaluation until all borders are noted to be clear of the tumor. This type of surgery has proven to be successful on skin in other areas of the body, particularly the face. It is currently being tried in several cancer treatment centers for superficial carcinoma of the vulva. Continuous follow-up is important for women who have had vulvar cancer, because areas of dystrophy and cancer can form in other parts of the vulva in the future.

In some women, particularly younger women or women who are immunosuppressed, such as women with HIV infection or those who have had organ transplants and are on immunosuppressant drugs, there seems to be a relationship between the human papilloma virus (HPV) infection of the skin and the development of cancer. To date, these relationships are statistical, and it is not clear whether or not the virus actually is involved in the cause of the cancer. Cancers in older women, however, are rarely associated with papilloma virus infection.

CASE STUDY

Sally is a seventy-two-year-old woman referred to me because of itching and burning of her vulva of two year's duration. She treated this herself with various creams that she purchased at the drugstore. These included vitamin A and D ointments and hydrocortisone cream. Although she got some relief at first, the itching always recurred, and with scratching she would often have some bloody discharge. She consulted her primary care physician about six months ago. He prescribed a stronger corticosteroid cream, which offered her some relief for a few months, but then the problem recurred worse than ever.

When I examined her, I noted that the skin of her vulva was very thin, with little pigmentation and no hair follicles. Her labia majora had just about disappeared, and her labia minora were very thin and flush with the vaginal opening. There were several areas that were quite thickened and white on her labia, and one included her clitoris. There were also a few areas between her vaginal opening and her rectum. Two areas, one on the left labia and one on the skin between the vagina and rectum, were quite thickened. After putting some xylocaine into the skin in these areas, I did punch biopsies, which were diagnosed as lichen sclerosis et atrophicus with areas of carcinoma in situ.

I then took Sally to the operating room and under anesthesia did a wide excision of the vulvar skin of the affected areas. After she healed and we received a

(continued)

CASE STUDY (CONTINUED)

pathology report indicating that all of the tumor had been removed and no area had been worse than carcinoma in situ, I prescribed for her 2 percent testosterone cream, the appropriate therapy for lichen sclerosis. She has been followed for the past two years and has done quite well.

Vaginal Cancer

The majority of vaginal cancers are also carcinomas of squamous cell origin developing in the superficial layers of the vagina. A rare exception is clear cell carcinoma of the vagina, which arises in islands of glandular cells isolated within the vagina during embryonic development in women who were exposed to diethylstilbestrol (DES) given to their mothers while they were embryos. This medication was used in the late 1940s and 1950s with the presumption that it prevented miscarriage. Even after it was found not to do so, it was used sporadically for other high-risk conditions until 1971. The discovery that it could be associated with the development of clear cell cancer of the vagina was reported in 1971, and the medication has not been used since in pregnancy. This means that there is a specific generation of women, the oldest of whom are now about fifty years old, who were exposed to this agent in utero and who need to be followed for the rest of their lives because of the potential for the development of clear cell cancer in those women who have the islands of glandular cells called adenosis. Clear cell cancer develops in 1 in 1,000 women with adenosis. Physicians examining patients annually who find nodules in the vagina in women who have had DES exposure should biopsy these to discovery clear cell cancer as early as possible.

The majority of vaginal cancers, however, are squamous cell cancers that are discovered because of vaginal bleeding or because of abnormalities noted on vaginal examination. Such areas should be biopsied so that the diagnosis can be made as early as possible. Treatment of vaginal carcinoma depends upon the extent of the disease and can be surgical, varying from a wide excision of the area to a complete removal of the vagina, or in the form of irradiation therapy. Fortunately, vaginal cancer is quite rare and can be diagnosed relatively early.

Cervical Cancer

Although cervical cancer is quite common in younger women, 41 percent of the annual deaths from cervical cancer occur in women over the age of sixty-five. Many cancers of the cervix in younger women arise from areas of dysplasia, a cellular change in the cervix that can progress to cancer in a small percentage of cases. Often, dysplasia stays unchanged for long periods of time or regresses. Cervical cancer in older women, however, often develops quite rapidly without going through the dysplastic stage. Screening is as important for older women as it is for younger women. One study estimates that women over the age of sixty-five could have a 63 percent improvement in five-year survival from this disease if they were given the benefit of regular screening. While 90 percent of the cervical cancers are of the squamous cell variety, about 10 percent arise from glandular cells within the cervical canal. Furthermore, whereas squamous cell carcinoma is related to a number of risk factors, including multiple sex partners, early onset of sexual activity, frequent pregnancies, and infections with the organisms that cause sexually transmitted diseases, adenocarcinoma occurs without these risk factors and equally in all age groups.

Recently, a relationship between the human papilloma virus (HPV) and cervical cancer has been noted on an epidemiologic basis. However, most older women do not demonstrate previous infection with HPV. Whether or not this lack of association also points to a different disease in older woman than in younger woman is not known. By and large, the development of squamous cell carcinoma in older women usually is more rapid, frequently without the other risk factors that have been noted.

Diagnosis of early cervical cancer is made by discovering an abnormality on Pap smear screening; by performing colposcopy, which is looking at the cervix closely with a specialized microscope called a colposcope that allows magnification of the cervical epithelium; and by discovering lesions after applying a substance called 3 percent acidic acid. The acidic acid causes dehydration of the cytoplasm of cells. Since dysplastic or cancer cells normally have very large nuclei and very small amounts of cytoplasm and are usually found to pile up on each other, the dysplastic or cancerous areas are often noted as white areas, called white epithelium. Because normal cervical epithelium consists of very large cells with very small nuclei, application of acidic acid causes no change in appearance. In addition, normal squamous epithelial cells are usually present in relatively few numbers and do not have the tendency to pile up as do dysplastic or cancer cells. The presence of a developing tumor calls upon the body to supply blood vessels, and these can be seen in the lesion through the microscope. Because the presence of white epithelium and evidence for developing small capillaries within the area indicates the development of a tumor, its presence is an indication for biopsy. As the tumor enlarges and becomes invasive, it may become more friable, and these newly formed blood vessels may be involved in bleeding from time to time. Therefore, a woman who experience bleeding between periods, particularly after intercourse, should be investigated for a cervical lesion.

Adenocarcinoma poses a somewhat different problem in diagnosis. Since the tumor arises from the cervical canal and often begins deep within the cervical glands, it may not shed cells that can be picked up on Pap smear at a very early period. Often the presence of atypical glandular cells is noted when the physician examines the canal with a cytobrush. Since malignant cells may not actually be seen with certainty, the diagnosis may be delayed. Physicians dealing with women who have such Pap smears must maintain a high index of suspicion and must biopsy the tissue of the canal as part of the colpsocopic examination. The colposcopy with biopsy and endocervical curettage is an office procedure and can be performed without anesthetic.

Recently, there has been a great deal of discussion about the frequency with which women should be screened with Pap smears. Most of this is based on economics. Currently the American College of Obstetricians and Gynecologists recommends annual screening for all high-risk women, that is, those who have the risk factors mentioned above; and at least every other year for women who have had three or more consecutive annual normal Pap smears and are monogamous. The ACOG guidelines leave the interval to the discretion of the physician, since the needs of each woman are different. Whether or not annual screening is cost effective for older women has not been determined. Given the rapidity and severity of developing cervical carcinoma in older women, I believe that annual screening should be performed.

The treatment of cervical cancer in its early stages is surgical. Carcinoma in situ, which is severe dysplasia in which the full thickness of the cervix is replaced by cancer cells but no invasion has taken place, can be treated with local excision called a cone biopsy. If the surgical margins at the endocervical canal and the vaginal portion of the cervix are clear of tumor following this procedure, the woman may simply be given follow-up Pap smears. For an older woman past menopause, a simple hysterectomy is also reasonable. This may be performed abdominally or vaginally, depending upon the other circumstances of her condition. Since cancer of the cervix spreads locally to surrounding tissue and to local lymph nodes, it has been shown that even minimally invasive tumors, that is, tumors that have not invaded for more than 3 mm below the basement membrane of the cervix, can also be treated with simple hysterectomy. This is because the local extent of the tumor is minimal and the lymph nodes are rarely involved. For a tumor localized to the cervix but more than just minimally invasive, the staging is Stage I, and a radical hysterectomy with pelvic lymph node dissection is appropriate. Stage I tumors have tumor in the local lymph nodes in about 15 percent of cases. For larger tumors that have spread from the cervix to the upper vagina and the tissue surrounding the uterus and cervix, the chances of lymph node spread is greater, and these individuals are usually treated with radiation therapy in the form of both radium or cesium implants and external beam therapy. Even with many of these larger lesions, cure can be obtained in a large number of cases. Needless to say, women who have been treated either surgically or with irradiation need to be followed with Pap smear screening in the future to ensure that recurrence does not take place.

CASE STUDY

Angela is a sixty-nine-year-old woman who is married and has had two children. She has no history of sexually transmitted diseases or multiple partners. On a recent health maintenance visit to her internist, her Pap smear was reported as atypical because of abnormal-appearing glandular cells. No obvious lesions were seen on the examination of her cervix. I performed an endocervical curettage and an endometrial biopsy to detect whether or not the abnormal cells could be coming from the cervix or endometrial cavity. Her endometrial biopsy simply showed atrophic endometrium, which is what would be expected for a woman of her age who is not on estrogen replacement therapy. The endocervical biopsy showed sheets of atypical-appearing glandular cells suggestive of carcinoma. After I performed a cone biopsy of her cervix under anesthesia, I noted a small adenocarcinoma with minimal invasion. Even though the cervical margins were free of tumor, I performed a vaginal hysterectomy and fortunately noted no other areas of tumor. Angela was fortunate to have had a tumor picked up early by Pap smear and biopsy, and her treatment was of necessity not extensive.

Endometrial Cancer

Endometrial cancer is usually seen in women who are past menopause and is rare in women before the menopause. The peak incidence is between the ages of fifty and seventy, but it can occur in older women as well. There seems to be two types of endometrial cancer. The first is related to excessive estrogen and was seen quite commonly during the 1970s, when estrogen was prescribed widely for postmenopausal women and in large doses. During that time, progesterone was not routinely used to counteract the effects of estrogen on the lining of the uterus. In general, large doses of estrogen over prolonged periods of time without progesterone counteraction will frequently lead to hyperplasia of the endometrium and, in some cases, to cancer. Some women produce a large amount of estrogen, which will cause the same reaction in the endometrium. This is seen particularly in obese women, because fat cells will convert androgens coming from the adrenal gland into estrogen. The endometrial cancer that is related to estrogen excess is generally a well-differentiated cell type, discovered early because of postmenopausal bleeding problems, and curable by simple hysterectomy.

The second type of endometrial cancer arises without the influence of estrogen but can certainly occur in women who are taking estrogen as a coincidental condition. This is usually a much more serious cell type that tends to progress more rapidly and has a lower cure rate. This type of cancer often requires both hysterectomy and further therapy with irradiation and chemotherapy.

Endometrial cancer seems to occur more commonly in women who have never had children but less commonly in women who have used birth control pills. In fact, the use of birth control pills during the reproductive years will cut the lifetime risk of endometrial cancer in half and make it about equal to the risk to women who have had five or more children.

Pap smears are not a good way to screen for endometrial cancer. They pick up only about 50 percent of the cancers, and unfortunately these are usually more advanced by the time they begin to shed abnormal cells. On the other hand, such cancers have a tendency to cause vaginal bleeding early in their development, so postmenopausal vaginal bleeding should be evaluated, usually by an endometrial biopsy. There are currently several ways to evaluate the endometrium in a postmenopausal woman. The first is by endometrial biopsy or dilation and curettage (D&C). While D&Cs have been performed commonly in the past, it has been shown that endometrial sampling with a biopsy instrument is just as effective in detecting endometrial cancer. Diagnosis from both a D&C and an endometrial biopsy is about 90 to 95 percent accurate.

Another way of screening the endometrium of a postmenopausal woman is to perform an ultrasound to measure the thickness of the endometrium. In general, cancers have not been seen when the endometrium is measured on both sides of the endometrial cavity, and does not exceed 5 mm. Women taking estrogen may have a thicker endometrium but may not require a biopsy unless bleeding is also present or the thickening is greater than 8 mm.

At times, older women develop endometrial polyps that are benign but may cause bleeding or distort the endometrium. By placing some saline into the endometrial cavity and performing a vaginal ultrasound examination, the physician may be able to see these abnormal structures. If abnormal structures are found or if the woman has a negative endometrial biopsy and continues to bleed, a hysteroscopic examination should be carried out. This is the placement of a small fiber-optic endoscope through the endocervical canal into the uterine cavity. There are instruments that can be utilized in the physician's office for diagnostic purposes. Other instruments can be utilized under anesthesia to allow the physician to actually operate in the endometrial cavity and perform biopsies and other procedures, such as excision of polyps. Today, D&Cs are rarely performed blindly and are almost always part of a hysteroscopic procedure.

The treatment for endometrial cancer depends upon the cell type, the depth of invasion of the tumor into the myometrium (muscle layer), the size of the uterus, and evidence for spread to other organs. Endometrial cancer frequently spreads through the lymphatic system, and it also spreads through the peritoneal cavity, probably by exiting the uterus through the fallopian tubes. Metastases may be found in distant areas such as lungs, the liver, the bone, and even the brain. Metastases are often found on peritoneal surfaces within the abdominal cavity and in the ovaries. Occasionally the tumor extends to the cervix, which then may allow metastases to pelvic lymph nodes. The tumor must then be treated as if it were a cervical cancer with either a radical hysterectomy or a hysterectomy plus pelvic X ray.

If the tumor is well differentiated and limited to the inner third of the myometrium, and the uterus is small without any evidence of spread to other organs (as seen by X ray or biopsy), a simple hysterectomy with removal of the ovaries will usually suffice. If the tumor has a poor cell type, is more deeply invaded into the uterus, is extensive in an enlarged uterus, or has spread to different sites, then a combination of surgery with chemotherapy or irradiation is usually indicated. The prognosis becomes poorer as the tumor is noted to be of poor cell type, large size, or distant spread. Clearly, early detection is important in order to have the best outcome. Thus, all evidence of vaginal bleeding after menopause should be investigated immediately and therapy instituted as soon as possible.

After a woman has been treated for endometrial cancer, she should be followed closely for many years, as recurrences have been noted ten to fifteen years after the initial tumor.

CASE STUDY

Harriet is a fifty-seven-year-old attorney who has been a judge for several years. She never married, never had children, but did take estrogen replacement hormone therapy after her menopause at age fifty-two. For the past five years, she has taken a combination estrogen/progesterone regimen and has had no vaginal bleeding. For the past three weeks she had had some spotting and some pinkish fluid discharge.

When she consulted me, I performed an endometrial biopsy, which was reported as an adenocarcinoma of the endometrium, Class II. (Class I endometrial lesions are well differentiated, Class II are intermediate, and Class III are

(continued)

CASE STUDY (CONTINUED)

poorly differentiated.) Since she had a normal-sized uterus and the rest of her evaluation was negative, I performed a total abdominal hysterectomy and bilateral removal of her ovaries and fallopian tubes. Although histologically the lesion was of intermediate maturity, it was quite small and localized to the lining of the uterus, leaving her prognosis quite good. She will be followed closely for several years.

OVARIAN CANCER

Ovarian cancer is a serious problem in women of all ages, but the incidence increases with age and reaches its highest risk by the age of eighty. Also, ovarian cancer occurring in women past age sixty-five is associated with a shorter period of survival. One study showed a mean survival of twenty-four months for older women, compared to more than four years for younger women. The women studied had advanced stage disease. Unfortunately, early disease is silent and is only picked up by chance during a pelvic examination demonstrating an enlarged ovary, on an ultrasound examination for another purpose, or at an operation for another purpose. Certainly, for old and young women alike, early detection offers the best chance of cure. Over a lifetime, a woman has about a 1 in 89 chance of developing ovarian cancer. This risk has encouraged physicians to remove the ovaries in women who are approaching menopause when they are undergoing a hysterectomy for other reasons. Some tumors of the peritoneal surface that occur on the ovaries also can occur in other parts of the peritoneal cavity. Removing the ovary does not remove the opportunity for this to happen, but it does lower the chance for developing cancer of the ovary. The decision whether or not to remove ovaries in a premenopausal woman certainly should be made by the patient and the physician together, considering the number of years of ovarian function that may be left and the risk of cancer in the particular woman. However, after menopause, there is little reason to keep the ovaries when a woman is to undergo a hysterectomy, and removal should be recommended.

Since there are no symptoms early in the disease, when a woman does become symptomatic, she usually has advanced disease. The symptoms that are often associated with carcinoma of the ovary are: bowel complaints, increased abdominal girth due to fluid and tumor accumulation in the peritoneal cavity, and abdominal pain. As the disease progresses, if it is not treated, bowel obstruction and symptoms associated with it may occur. A woman will generally report a decrease in appetite and may report loss of appetite, decreased calorie intake, and weight loss in spite of increasing abdominal girth.

The majority of ovarian tumors in older women are cystic in nature and appear to have multiple cysts on ultrasound. The cell type is usually serous cystadenocarcinoma or mucinous cystadenocarcinoma, but a variety of other solid and cystic tumors, some of which may produce estrogen or other hormones, are possible. The cancer marker CA-125 has been reported to rise in the blood of women with serous cystadenocarcinomas. Unfortunately, this is not a specific marker and is often elevated in other conditions such as endometriosis, fibroids, and other types of tumors. Also, it does not tend to be elevated in mucinous cystadenocarcinomas, which are seen fairly frequently in older women. It is not a good screening indicator and will only be present when the tumor is already present and growing. It does have a value in following patients after treatment who have had serous cystadenocarcinomas, since recurrence will often be heralded by an increase in this cancer marker.

Prognosis for ovarian cancer depends on the cell type of the tumor and the stage of the tumor. If the tumor can be caught early while it is still limited to one or both ovaries and has not spread to the peritoneal cavity, the cure rate can be quite high. However, as the tumor spreads, the cure rate is reduced.

Treatment has two primary approaches. In the surgical approach, the tumor is debulked as much as possible. The patient will have a large vertical incision made in her abdomen and will undergo a total hysterectomy, with removal of both ovaries and tubes. She will have sampling of her peritoneum from several different areas of her peritoneal cavity and also have sampling of her abdominal lymph nodes. She will undergo the excision of as much as possible of her omentum, the apron of tissue that is draped over the peritoneal cavity from the stomach and that generally contains fat cells and lymph nodes. Since this is a frequent site of tumor extension, as much of it as possible is removed. A physician will also inspect the areas above the liver and below the dome of the diaphragm, as this is often a spot to which the tumor extends and hides. All tumor that can removed is removed surgically with the of leaving less than 2 grams of tumor present in the peritoneal cavity. The reason for this is that good chemotherapeutic agents are now available for treatment of ovarian cancer and are most effective when the tumor bulk is small. Patients who have advanced stage carcinoma of the ovary are then given several courses of chemotherapy. Although this has changed through the years, today the use of agents containing platinum (such as cisplatinum) and Taxol are currently in use. Even in advanced disease it is possible for patients to survive from five to ten years with adequate therapy, and this is certainly worth doing. Unfortunately, older women have often not been offered such therapy and therefore have been deprived of both a longer life and perhaps a good quality of life.

Ovarian cancer seems to occur more frequently in women who have not had children or who have had very few children and is reduced in women who used birth control pills during their reproductive years. In fact, prolonging the use of birth control pills often reduces the risk of ovarian cancer by two thirds. It is thought that the risk of ovarian cancer is related to frequency of ovulation in that both pregnancy and birth control pills limit the number of ovulation events and therefore may reduce the risk of ovarian cancer later.

Women who have been treated for ovarian cancer require close follow-up for the rest of their lives.

CASE STUDY

Marge was a seventy-five-year-old woman who enjoyed good health until about three months previously. At that time, she noted that her abdomen was somewhat enlarged and her dresses felt tight. She thought she was putting on weight and compensated by wearing looser-fitting clothing. However, the condition continued to get worse. She noted some abdominal cramping, constipation, and loss of appetite.

When she came in for consultation, upon physical examination, she was found to have palpable masses throughout her abdomen as well as evidence of fluid in her abdomen. A chest X ray showed fluid in her chest. When some of this was tapped off, a bloody fluid was obtained and upon histologic section, cancer cells were found to be present.

Marge was referred to a gynecologic oncologist, who performed her surgery and discovered an advanced serous cystadenocarcinoma of the ovary. A debulking operation was carried out, and Marge was treated with chemotherapy. Although her lesion was quite advanced, she has survived for four years but has required subsequent courses of chemotherapy and a second debulking operation during this time period.

Even with advanced cancer of the ovary, today's treatments can offer the patient prolongation of life and reasonable comfort. Before aggressive management of such cancers, Marge would not have been treated and would have died within a very short period of time.

OTHER CANCERS

Tumors of the lymphatic system, such as lymphomas, leukemias, and tumors of the urinary tract, also occur relatively frequently in older women. Thus, any abnormal growth or lump noted should be immediately biopsied. Lymphomas may occur in any organ of the body and will often grow quite rapidly. While surgical excision is useful in some lymphomas, depending upon where they are located, the treatment is primarily chemotherapy, with or without irradiation. There are many successful protocols that can offer patients with lymphomas an opportunity either for cure or at least for increased survival.

Leukemias often cause increased tiredness, weakness, and a general poor feeling overall. Because the leukemia is a cancer of the bone marrow, and the bone marrow produces red blood cells, white blood cells, and platelets, the symptoms may relate to anemia because of an impingement on red cell production, infection because of interference with white blood cell production, or bleeding because of interruption in platelet production. Symptoms related to these should certainly be investigated. Often the diagnosis of leukemia is made with a simple blood test, usually followed by a bone marrow evaluation. The likelihood of a chronic leukemia in an older person is greater than the likelihood of an acute leukemia. Both respond, in many instances, to chemotherapy, which offers patients a chance for a cure or for prolonged survival.

Tumors of the urinary tract usually are first discovered after a person finds blood in the urine (hematuria), or experiences obstructive signs or pain, or because of metastases to other structures. Occasionally, tumors of the kidney metastasize quite early to bone and cause pain before they manifest themselves with symptoms related to the urinary tract itself. People who experience any of these findings should be investigated for tumors of the kidneys or bladder.

CONCLUSION

The best way to cure cancer is to detect it early or to prevent it altogether. Some tumors can be prevented by early screening or by careful observation of symptoms and findings. The detection of cancer is a responsibility of both women and their physicians. Denial of symptoms on either part can lead to advanced disease. Therefore, it is wise to use whatever screening methods are available, to have frequent medical evaluations, and to report any abnormal symptoms as soon as they occur. For many cancers, the diagnosis does not have to be a death sentence. Even when cancers cannot be cured, it may be possible to prolong life, and maintain a good quality of life, with early detection and proper treatment.

CHAPTER 12

Benign Pelvic Tumors; Fibroids, Cysts, and Other Lumps and Bumps

Many benign tumors and cysts can arise in pelvic organs. Because they are benign, they are usually not life threatening. The problem arises from the fact that when they are detected by pelvic or abdominal examination or by some imaging study such as ultrasound, it is usually not known whether they are indeed benign. Therefore, their discovery generally leads to more tests and often surgery. This chapter discusses the types of problems that can occur and also the kinds of dilemmas that such tumors can cause with respect to diagnosis and treatment. In general, these are not tumors that will cause death, but they may cause discomfort or other local problems because of their growth and size.

BENIGN TUMORS OF THE UTERUS

Two types of benign tumors occur in the uterus. The first are endometrial polyps, which grow from the lining of the uterus (endometrium) into the cavity of the uterus. These can become quite large and generally cause bleeding fairly early on. They can often be seen by ultrasound and can be identified and removed through the hystero-scope. Many patients with endometrial polyps become very anemic, and because of the heavy bleeding they believe they have cancer. While it is not possible to differen-tiate those polyps that may contain malignancies from benign ones on ultrasound examination, hysteroscopic removal both removes the polyp, thereby curing the problem, and allows the pathologist to make a tissue diagnosis to definitely rule out malignance. If a malignancy is found in a polyp, the further treatment will be deter-mined by whether or not the base of the polyp or the rest of the endometrium is involved. If it is, a hysterectomy and other treatment as is necessary could be called for. If, however, the malignant change is present only in the tip of the polyp and not in its stalk, removal is all that is necessary.

Vaginal bleeding in a woman past the menopause who is not taking hormone replacement therapy is always frightening. However, only about one third of these women will actually have hyperplasia of the endometrium or cancer. The other two thirds many of whom will have polyps of the endometrium, will have benign lesions.

The other benign condition that can cause a mass or masses arising from the uterus is fibroids. The technical term for these is leiomyomata. Although they are common, occurring in about 40 percent of women before menopause, they tend to shrink and become very small after menopause unless the woman continues to take fairly high doses of estrogen replacement. In a study of 87 patients with pelvic masses over the age of 51, who were followed at St. Luke's-Roosevelt Hospital in New York City, 22 were found to have fibroids of the uterus. Nineteen of these were between the ages of 51 and 60 and 3 between the ages of 61 and 70. No fibroids were detected in women over the age of 70. In contrast, 24 of the 87 women had benign cysts of the ovary, 28 turned out to have cancer in the pelvis, and 4 surprisingly had benign cystic teratomas (dermoid cysts), which are usually seen in younger women. One of these actually occurred in a woman past the age of 70. Two of the women were found to have endometriomas of the ovaries (endometriosis), and 7 had various and sundry miscellaneous masses that happen to be present in the pelvis. While fibroids are a real possibility, particularly in women who are not very far past menopause, they must be differentiated from other tumors in the pelvis, many of which are benign.

Fibroids are almost always benign. Leiomyosarcoma, a malignant form, does occur about once in every two hundred cases of fibroids. Therefore, solid masses of the uterus that persist past menopause or may seem to be growing should be removed. Even when this is done, most of these masses will turn out to be benign.

BENIGN TUMORS OF THE OVARY

Tumors of the ovary are classified with tumors of the adnexae. The adnexae consist of the ovaries, the fallopian tubes, and the structures in the mesentery (connective tissue) that exist between them. Although the chance of malignancy in cysts and solid masses of the adnexae increases with age, the majority will still be benign at a ratio of usually about 2 to 1. So, if your physician discovers a cyst, it does not mean you have a cancer. When an adnexal mass is discovered, a physician usually orders an ultrasound. This allows the physician to determine whether or not the mass is solid or cystic. If it is cystic, ultrasound can determine whether it is a simple cyst, that is, a cyst with only one cavity, or whether it is a complex cyst, with multiple compartments and possibly solid components. It also allows the physician to determine whether or not there is any free fluid in the peritoneal cavity. The presence of fluid, termed ascites, and the finding of a multiloculated (multicompartment) cyst, increase the chances but certainly do not make it definite that the lesion is malignant. In a Pittsburgh study of 150 tumors of the adnexae in women past the age of fifty, 103 proved to be benign and 47 malignant. Size was important in this and other studies. In tumors less than 5 cm, only one proved to be malignant. The larger the tumor, the more likely it was to be malignant, but even in fairly large tumors, some were still benign. There are several types of ovarian tumors. Of those that are solid, that is, they do not contain any cystic areas, the fibromas are still the most common, and these are benign. Fibromas may grow to be very large, and because of their effect on the lymphatic system, they may actually be associated with fluid in the abdomen and chest. Removing the tumor cures the patient.

The first abdominal surgical operation reported in the United States occurred in 1809 in Kentucky. A physician named Ephraim McDowell removed a huge fibroma from a woman's abdomen on the kitchen table without anesthesia. (It was reported that she recited the Psalms while the operation was carried out.) The woman went on to live a long full life.

Some fibroids of the uterus arising from the outer portion of the uterus on stalks masquerade as adnexal tumors. In the Pittsburgh study, ten of the 150 tumors proved to be fibroids ranging in size from less than 5 cm to over 10 cm.

There are other solid tumors of the ovary that are usually benign. Some produce hormones, and if these are androgens (male sex hormones), the woman may note masculinizing symptoms such as deepening voice, atrophy of the breasts, and hair growth. If the hormones are estrogen, which is more often the case, the woman may begin to menstruate once again. While many of these are benign tumors, a few are malignant and need to be evaluated carefully for this possibility.

Cystic tumors of the ovary are more common. They generally arise from the covering of the ovary, known as the epithelium. In both the malignant and the benign form, these may vary in size. In the Pittsburgh study, 53 of the 150 tumors proved to be benign epithelial cystic tumors, and 33 proved to be malignant. The benign tumors varied in size from less than 5 cm to greater than 10 cm, but the malignant tumors were almost all larger than 10 cm.

An occasional histologic variation of cancer are the so-called borderline tumors. These tumors resemble malignancies but are usually localized to the ovary and have a very slow growing potential. Most are cured by removing the ovary, but some do progress over a long period of time. Four borderline tumors were discovered among the 150 women with adnexal masses in the Pittsburgh study. Two were between 5 and 10 cm in diameter, and two were greater than 10 cm in diameter. Eight of the tumors in the Pittsburgh study were from nonovarian structures of the adnexae. These are usually cysts arising from embryonic remnants and are designated, as a group, as paraovarian cysts. They are benign but can become quite large.

Other studies have demonstrated findings similar to those reported in the Pittsburgh study. The important thing to remember is that the finding of a pelvic mass, even a fairly large mass in an older woman, does not necessarily mean a malignancy. In general, the older the patient and the larger the mass, the more likely it is to be a malignant lesion. But even in the larger lesions in older woman, benign lesions still occur.

While the presence of a pelvic mass generally leads to further evaluation, and often to surgery, not all masses need to be treated this way. If the physician is fairly sure that the mass is a solid tumor arising from the uterus, it can be observed. If it is a fibroid, it will probably continue to regress in size as the woman gets older. The general rule would be to observe it, following the woman every three months with pelvic examination and, if the size cannot accurately be determined in this fashion, with ultrasound examinations. Tumors that are becoming smaller can be watched. Tumors that are getting larger should be removed. For a postmenopausal woman with an enlarging uterine mass, a hysterectomy is the best course of action.

But what about cysts? Simple cysts, less than 5 cm in diameter in older woman, can be followed. I have followed women into their eighties with 4 to 5 cm simple cysts that do not change. Clearly, if they are enlarging or if they contain multiple cysts, they should be removed.

One dilemma is the complex cystic mass without solid components that is probably a benign serous cystadenoma. There is some debate as to whether or not these should be removed if they are small. We do not know whether or not such lesions become malignant with time, and it is probably prudent to remove them. Clearly, those larger than 5 cm in size should be removed.

In dealing with cystic adnexal masses, the physician will generally order a CA-125 assay prior to surgery. Many benign lesions will cause a moderate elevation of the CA-125 assay. If the lesion proves to be malignant, this is a good way of following certain types of tumors. CA-125 assay is a good marker for the prognosis of serous cystadenocarcinoma but is not a good marker for other types of tumors, such as mucinous cystadenocarcinoma. As time goes on, other tumor markers will probably be discovered that may be helpful in following women with other types of tumors. These lesions present a dilemma for patients and physicians.

CASE STUDY

Kate is an eighty-year-old, healthy, active woman. She is the widow of a corporate executive. She and her husband were in the habit of going to the Mayo Clinic once a year for complete evaluations. He died five years ago of a sudden heart attack. Since she had the means, she continued to visit the Mayo Clinic annually for her evaluations. When she was seventy-six, a 4 to 5 cm cystic mass of her right ovary was noted. Ultrasound showed this to be a simple cyst, and the possibilities of malignancy were discussed with her. Her physician at the Mayo Clinic advised surgical removal, but she elected not to have this done.

Four years later, she consulted me for an annual evaluation. I could palpate the adnexal mass on pelvic examination but did an ultrasound, just to be sure. The mass was still 4 to 5 cm and still a simple cyst. We decided to continue to follow it. She is currently eighty-eight and still in good health, and her mass is unchanged.

This cyst is most likely a serous cystadenoma, which is a benign lesion, and it is certainly not growing. Since I had the advantage of a four-year history when Kate first consulted me, I felt it was quite safe to continue to follow her, and nothing has changed.

CASE STUDY

Evelyn's is a different story. She had had a vaginal hysterectomy and pelvic repair for a prolapsed uterus at age forty-nine. As is common with a vaginal hysterectomy, the surgeon had left her ovaries intact. She had seen me for annual check

(continued)

CASE STUDY (CONTINUED)

ups for the past five years. At age sixty-two, she was discovered to have a 10 cm cystic mass of her right ovary that had not been present the year before. The workup showed no obvious metastatic spread and no fluid (ascites) in the pelvic cavity. A gynecological oncologist and I operated on her and removed both ovaries. Her right ovary was replaced by a 10 cm cystic mass, and the left ovary was small and benign. We performed a staging operation, which consisted of removal of many lymph nodes in her peritoneal cavity and a partial removal of her omentum. When we were finished, there was no evidence of tumor in her abdominal cavity, and the histology of the tumor was reported as a borderline tumor of the right ovary. Evelyn was discussed at the tumor conference, and it was decided not to offer her chemotherapy because of the borderline nature of her tumor. This is the usual management for such tumors.

Evelyn was followed with pelvic examinations, laboratory studies, and a CA-125 assay at regular intervals and did well for six years. In her seventh year, her CA-125 assay suddenly began to rise by relatively small increments. The rise continued for two consecutive months, and she was subjected to a reevaluation and found to have a few small pelvic masses noted by CT scan. She was reevaluated and reoperated, and she was found to have metastatic disease in the lymph nodes within her peritoneal cavity. Again, the histology was reported as borderline tumor, but because of the metastatic disease, Evelyn was treated with chemotherapy. Following a total course of chemotherapy, the tumor disappeared, and she again was followed with routine examinations and CA-125 assays. Three years later, the assays again began to rise. She was again reevaluated. This time she had considerable tumor in her peritoneal cavity and involving her bowel. Although she was treated with subsequent courses of chemotherapy, her course now was rapidly downhill, and she died a year and a half after the second recurrence and ten and a half years after her tumor was first discovered. By this time, she was almost seventy-four years old.

This is a fairly typical story for a woman with the occasional borderline tumor that recurs. Some hormone-producing benign ovarian tumors lead to cancer of the uterus.

CASE STUDY

Linda was fifty-six years old and five years postmenopausal when she began to have heavy vaginal bleeding. On evaluation she was found to have a slightly enlarged uterus and a well-differentiated adenocarcinoma of the endometrium. She was also found to have a 6 cm firm left ovarian mass that, on ultrasound, proved to be solid. She underwent a total abdominal hysterectomy and had both ovaries removed. Her right ovary was benign, but the left ovary was replaced by
(continued)

CASE STUDY (CONTINUED)

a solid tumor, which proved to be a thecoma, a tumor arising from ovarian stromal cells that produce large amounts of estrogen hormone. The estrogen probably stimulated the uterus to the point that it developed a cancer of the endometrium. It was a histologically well-differentiated cancer, which indicates a less aggressive tumor and the patient has done well for the past five years without any evidence of recurrence. At this point it is likely that she is cured.

This is a typical story of an estrogen-secreting tumor that has probably hyperstimulated the uterus into going through cancer changes. It does not always cause cancer. Frequently the bleeding occurs before this has happened, but in Linda's case, it had gone that far. Thecomas are not very common, but they do occur in combination with heavy vaginal bleeding, in this case related to carcinoma of the uterus. An adnexal mass tips off the diagnosis.

OTHER PELVIC TUMORS

The pelvis is rich in blood vessels, lymph nodes, and connective tissue. In addition, the bladder, urethra, colon, and rectum are also present in the pelvis. Therefore, many nongynecologic tumors may arise from these pelvic structures. With respect to blood vessels and the lymphatic system, a variety of possibilities can occur. Aneurysms (protruding areas of weakness in a blood vessel wall) of pelvic arteries may present as pelvic masses, and tumors of the lymphoid system such as lymphomas also frequently present in the pelvis. Tumors of nerve origin such as neurofibromas are possible. They are frequently seen in conjunction with a condition known as von Recklinghausen's disease, or neurofibromatosis. This is a familial condition transmitted as an autosomal dominant, meaning that half the children will have the disease if either parent is affected. Because it is autosomal dominant (only one gene of a pair is affected) there are frequently new mutations in the affected gene, giving rise to the disease. Someone may have neurofibromatosis without either parent being affected, but the affected person will pass the disease along to half of his or her offspring. These are frequently solid tumors arising from nerve sheaths, and the pelvis is a fairly common place for them to occur, although they are usually multiple throughout the body.

The fibrous connective tissue of the pelvis may give rise to fibromas and occasionally fibrosarcomas, the malignant version of fibroma.

Bladder tumors may occur, many of which are benign, and diverticulitis of the colon as well as polyps of the rectum or colon may also occur. Diverticulitis is a condition in which an outpouching or diverticulum of the colon may become inflamed and infected, causing an inflammatory mass. It is often difficult to differentiate this from cancer of the bowel, and occasionally these masses will rupture, causing pelvic abscess and peritonitis. Diverticulitis as well as colon and rectal polyps will usually become recognized because of gastrointestinal symptoms and possibly rectal bleeding.

CONCLUSIONS

Pelvic tumors are common. They can arise from several structures, can have several different symptoms ranging from none to symptoms involving other organ systems, and they are usually worrisome for the woman and her physician. A diagnosis must be made. At times it can be made by laboratory tests and imaging procedures such as ultrasound and CT scan, but often the diagnosis must be made by observing the tumor directly via either laparoscopy (the placement of an endoscope into the abdomen) or laparotomy (the surgical operning of the abdomen) and with a biopsy to obtain a tissue diagnosis. Removal of the organs is usually dictated either by inability to determine whether the tumor is malignant at the time of surgery, or because the tumor itself is causing local symptoms. Some tumors have malignant potential, but in most cases it is just about impossible to determine which tumor will move from a benign to malignant state over time. Malignant tumors are probably malignant from the beginning, and benign tumors probably remain benign, but this is certainly not definite according to our current knowledge. It is best to bring all unusual symptoms and findings to the attention of your physician. It is important to be sure that a proper diagnosis is made, and if there is any doubt the tumor should be removed. If there is doubt it is always more prudent to remove the tumor and be sure than to watch and worry. Small tumors can be removed via the laparoscope, but if there is fear that the condition may be malignant, it is best to perform a laparotomy so that proper evaluation and staging can take place. The decision of how to approach a problem surgically must be individualized for each woman and her needs and only after a frank discussion of the options between the woman and her doctor.

CHAPTER 13

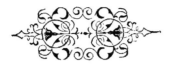

Vulvar and Vaginal Irritations and Discomfort

With aging, the skin of the vulva and the epithelium (lining) of the vagina become thinner. Much of this is due to the loss of estrogen and is seen to a lesser degree in women who take estrogen replacement therapy. In addition to the thinning of the various layers of the vulvar skin and a loss of elasticity of the subepithelial (dermis) portion of the skin, the changes with aging also involve a decrease in subcutaneous fatty tissue and shrinking of the labia. In much older women the labia will nearly disappear and the vaginal opening will be flush with the perineum, losing the usual texture and characteristic of the vulva. The pubic hair usually becomes very scant, may turn gray or white, or may disappear entirely, and with a loss of elasticity of the skin, varicose veins may appear on the vulva. As the skin thins, small blood vessels may be noticed at or near the surface, and as the skin of the vulva becomes more friable, bleeding may occur.

As the vaginal epithelium thins, the tissue of the vagina beneath the epithelium loses its elasticity, and there is a tendency for the vaginal tube to narrow. Since the epithelium is dependent on estrogen, if estrogen is not replaced, it will become thin, and the surface cells that are normally squamous cell type will be replaced by basal cells, cells of the lower level of the tissue. Normally the vaginal epithelium contains a good deal of glycogen, which nourishes the lactobacilli normally present and keeps the vaginal pH on the acid side. This acidity helps to prevent infections, particularly with organisms such as yeast. With the epithelial changes and the loss of glycogen, the lactobacilli also disappear, allowing an increased growth of other bacteria, often giving rise to a watery, fishy-smelling discharge called atrophic vaginitis. At the same time, normal lubrication of the vagina disappears, and vaginal dryness or cracking may occur. Intercourse may be uncomfortable, and cracking of the vaginal epithelium and skin of the vulva related to intercourse may occur. This may cause soreness, irritation, and bleeding.

At this time, the symptoms of atrophic vaginitis can be relieved with estrogen taken by mouth or patch or used in the form of vaginal cream. Although vaginally applied estrogen will be absorbed into the circulation, it is possible to have a positive effect, reversing the symptoms of atrophic vaginitis even when a small amount of vaginal estrogen is used every other night or twice a week. The amount of absorption taking place will then be much less than what would occur with the oral use of estrogen. There are several vaginal estrogen preparations available, including vaginal creams of Premarin, Estrace, and Ogen. Estrogen cream improves the thickness of epithelium of the vagina, stimulates the production of protective squamous cells, increases the amount of glycogen storage, and therefore stimulates the return of the lactobacilli. These corrections usually eliminate the bacterial overgrowth and reverse the symptoms. It is then important to keep up the vaginal estrogen therapy on a twice-a-week basis.

There is still quite a controversy about whether or not women who ordinarily could not take estrogen replacement therapy can use vaginal estrogen. Basically, given the symptoms that women suffer with atrophic vaginitis, and the fact the blood levels of estrogen will be quite low with this type of estrogen replacement, most women can probably utilize this therapy.

The thinning of vulvar skin, the loss of subepithelial fat, and the shrinking of the labia may only be partially reversed by local estrogen therapy. In most cases, these areas respond best to oral estrogen. But in women who have a contraindication to the use of systemic estrogen, it is probably reasonable to try a low-dose local therapy.

EFFECT OF TAMOXIFEN ON VULVAR SKIN AND VAGINAL EPITHELIUM

Many women being treated for breast cancer take tamoxifen for up to five years. Tamoxifen is a weak estrogen that acts as an agonist and an antagonist. This means that in some situations it behaves as estrogen, and in other situations it acts as an antiestrogen. The usual dose of tamoxifen taken by women being treated for breast cancer is 20 mg a day. This amount has been shown to improve epithalization of the vagina in postmenopausal women, although in women who are premenopausal, the results may be just the opposite. In postmentopausal women, tamoxifen lowers the vaginal pH, retards vaginal atrophy, and increases the squamous epithelium covering of the vagina. In some postmenopausal women, however, it has been associated with a thinning of the vulvar skin and a subsequent increase in discomfort.

VULVAR DYSTROPHIES

Vulvar dystrophies are changes in the skin of the vulva that are nonneoplastic in nature. Some, however, are related to later neoplastic change. The current classification of these nonneoplastic epithelial disorders of the vulvar skin are 1) squamous cell hyperplasia, 2) lichen sclerosis, and 3) others.

Squamous Cell Hyperplasia

It is not definitely known what cause squamous cell hyperplasia, but it may be due to chronic moisture in the area of the vulva, leading to itching and scratching. Over time, the epithelium thickens, and there is frequently an inflammatory reaction noted in the subepithelial area (dermis). Some areas appear quite grossly thickened and should be biopsied to rule out precancerous or cancerous changes.

Treatment consists of keeping the skin dry, removing potential allergens such as soaps, deodorants, or the use of scented toilet papers from the area, treating vaginal discharges and infections, and applying corticosteroid creams. One-percent hydrocortisone cream purchased as an over-the-counter medication can be used, but often a more powerful corticosteroid medication should be prescribed by a physician. This approach to therapy will tend to stop the itching and therefore the itching/scratching cycle. Corticosteroids, particularly the stronger types, should not be used for prolonged periods of time as they may cause thinning and atrophy of the vulvar skin. The important thing to remember in squamous cell hyperplasia is that areas that persist, seem thickened, and appear different from other areas of the skin should be biopsied. Squamous cell cancer can develop in such areas.

Lichen Sclerosis

This condition has had many names over the years, including lichen sclerosis, kraurosis, primary atrophy of the vulva, and atrophic leukoplakia. Currently, the term *lichen sclerosis* is used, and essentially it means the thinning of the epithelium and subepithelial (dermis) areas of the skin. It can occur in women of any age but is most common in the elderly. The complaints are usually itching, irritation, and, at times, stricture of the vulva area around the vaginal introitus. The skin appears parchmentlike, and the labia are usually grossly thinned. At times, the labia minora are stuck to the skin of the vulva. There may be areas of whitish epithelium. There is usually a decrease in pubic hair, and the labia may actually disappear. The clitoris may be fixed by adhesions beneath the clitoral hood. Biopsies should be taken of the thickened whitish areas as they may be precancerous in type, but for the most part this is a benign condition.

The primary treatment is 2 percent testosterone propionate cream. It should be used nightly or every other night until improvement is noted, then used twice a week for several years. Some women are allergic to the solvent base, and their pharmacist can put testosterone in a nonallergic base. Occasionally testosterone will cause an unwanted increase in libido in an elderly woman. In such situations, progesterone cream can be substituted. It is used twice a day since the half-life of progesterone is 5 1/2 hours. Corticosteroids can be used on a limited basis, with mild corticosteroids (0.5 to 1.0 percent hydrocortisone cream) preferred. In general the stronger corticosteroids will cause increased thinning of the skin and over time will make matters worse.

CASE STUDY

Jerri is a seventy-two-year-old woman who was referred to me because of itching, burning, and cracking of the skin between the posterior portion of her vagina and her rectum. Her physician had given her high doses of corticosteroid
(continued)

cream, which at first relieved her symptoms but after a while had no effect. She takes hormone replacement therapy and is otherwise in good health.

Upon examination, the vulva appeared very atrophic. There were very few pubic hairs noted, most of which were gray. The labia had about disappeared, and the vaginal opening was flush with the skin of the perineum. The skin of the vulva appeared very thin, and there were several white patches along each side of the vaginal opening. These were biopsied, and the pathology report was lichen sclerosis.

Jerri was prescribed 2 percent testosterone cream every night for four weeks. After that time there was improvement of both her symptoms and the appearance of her vulva. The white patches had almost disappeared, and the skin appeared more healthy and pink. She used testosterone cream nightly for one more month and then used twice-a-week applications. She will be seen at six-month intervals, primarily to ensure that no new lesions develop on her vulva and that she continues to be free of symptoms.

Other Dermatoses

There are a number of other vulvar skin disorders that can be lumped under this subheading. Each is different, and each requires different therapy. One such is allergic dermatitis, which also is associated with scratching and irritation but disappears when the allergen can be found. Appropriate therapy is bathing with a soap of neutral pH such as Neutrogena and avoiding detergents in the laundering of underwear and other clothes that will be coming in contact with the vulva. Feminine deodorants, scented toilet paper, and other skin creams should be avoided. If a specific allergen can be identified, it should be eliminated.Psoriasis is another fairly common skin condition that can affect the vulva. Generally, the woman has psoriasis in other parts of the body. This condition should be referred to a dermatologist for up-to-date management.

A number of other skin conditions of lesser or more serious natures can occur in the vulva as they can in other parts of the body and have various diagnoses and specific treatments. Any suspicious lesion of the vulva, persistent itching or burning, or other vulvar discomfort should be brought to the attention of a physician so that the correct diagnosis can be made and therapy instituted.

VAGINITIS

In older women the commonest form of vaginitis is atrophic vaginitis. However, older woman are just as susceptible to specific vaginal infections as are younger women. There are three basic types to consider: yeast vaginitis, trichamonas vaginitis, and bacterial vaginosis.

Yeast Vaginitis

The majority of yeast infections are caused by an organism called Candida albicans. There are other candida species, but they are less common. The symptoms of candida infection are irritation and inflammation of the vagina and vulva, burning and itching, frequently irritated by urination, and a thick cheesy white discharge (appearing like cottage cheese). The specific diagnosis can be made by a potassium hydroxide wet mount preparation in which the physician puts a small amount of the discharge into a drop of potassium hydroxide and views it under the microscope without any specific stain. Potassium hydroxide destroys all of the vaginal epithelial cells and bacteria but leaves the candida organisms, which are resistant, available to be seen under the microscope. These appear as long stringy organisms called hyphae on which there may be small budding structures that appear like small grapes on a vine. The organisms may also be cultured. In general, a diagnosis can be made from the KOH mount in conjunction with the symptom of the patient and the appearance of the vulva and vagina.

There are several choices of treatment. The first is a group of vaginal creams or suppositories that fit into the family imidazoles. The chemical names are clotrimazole, miconazole, terconazole, and butaconazole. Many of these are available over the counter and can be purchased without prescription as medications such as Monistat and GyneLotrimin. For women who have had such infections before and who have the signs and symptoms of a yeast infection again, therapy may be instituted without a trip to the to the doctor by purchasing one of these mediations. Probably 90 to 95 percent of attacks can be cured in this fashion. If the symptoms do not disappear or if the problem recurs, a physician should be consulted. It has recently been noted that women recovering from a yeast infection that has been treated often will note a return of symptoms. The tendency has always been to treat again, but many of the symptoms of the yeast infection in a resolving case are usually due to a continuing of the irritation caused by the infection and not by the infection itself. It is therefore useful to have a physician examine you if you are having an apparent recurrence. This is probably a good time for a culture. If the culture is negative and the epithelium of the vagina appears to be healthy, it is best not to retreat with an anticandida medicine, as it may simply prolong the symptoms. I have seen this over and over again in my practice and do use cultures to be sure the infection is cleared up.

Women who have recurrent yeast infections should be evaluated for some underlying cause. First of all, conditions that change the pH of the vagina and increase the amount of sugar in the vaginal tissue may contribute to recurrent yeast infections. Diabetes is a good example of this, and women with recurrent yeast infections should be evaluated for the possibility of diabetes mellitus.

Second, a decrease in immune status may also lead to yeast infections. This is seen in women who have HIV infections or in women who are on anti-immune therapy for organ transplants. A woman who suffers from recurrent yeast infections should be evaluated for the possibility of an HIV infection.

Many women seem susceptible to yeast infections in spite of having an apparently intact immune system and no evidence for diabetes mellitus. In this situation, the yeast organisms may be colonized in the GI tract, and clearing up the disease locally only puts off the next attack until new organisms can again invade the vagina. About 25 percent of women carry a yeast organism in their vagina as normal vaginal flora and only have symptoms when something occurs to change the component of bacteria in the vagina. An example of this is taking an antibiotic that may kill some of the usual vaginal flora, allowing the yeast to overgrow. When some women have to take an antibiotic, they can expect a yeast infection. These women should probably be given prophylactic yeast treatment when they take an antibiotic because of another illness. For women whose bowels are colonized, oral antiyeast medications are available. This situation should be assessed and diagnosed by a physician who will prescribe the oral medications if indicated.

CASE STUDY

Amanda is eighty years old. She has always been prone to yeast infections, but these have generally gone away with local antiyeast creams. She was seen because two attempts to eradicate her current infection with vaginal antiyeast medications had not worked. Her vulva was extremely edematous and red. The skin was cracked in several places, there was a white discharge, and she was extremely uncomfortable. A portion of the discharge was placed in a potassium hydroxide droplet, and evidence for yeast was noted. A culture eventually demonstrated a strong overgrowth of candida organisms. While Amanda has been in reasonably good health, she does weigh 250 pounds.

Because of the recurrent nature of her infection, the fact that it has not been eradicated, her weight, and the extreme symptomatology she was suffering, I elected to treat her with an oral antifungicidal medication, Difluocan, for seven days. I also suggested sitz baths with an Aveeno solution, which is an oatmeal preparation, and sent a blood sugar for evaluation to the laboratory.

Her blood sugar returned at 250, indicating diabetes mellitus. Her family physician was contacted, and after evaluating the patient further, began her on insulin and diet therapy. She required three courses of Difloucan therapy for one week each before the vulvovaginitis was brought under control and she was made comfortable. By this time, her diabetes was controlled. She has been followed for six months since this initial episode and has done well.

This severe case of recurrent vulvovaginitis occurred in an uncontrolled diabetic. Her therapy required both aggressive management of her yeast infection and control of her diabetes. Oatmeal sitz baths were used to give her local relief while the therapy was being carried out.

Trichomonas Vaginitis

Trichomonas vaginitis is usually found in young, sexually active women, but it may be seen in sexually active older women or in older women who have come in contact with this organism through contact with others who are infected. The organism is not a bacterium but rather is a protozoan, a one-cell animal. The symptoms are severe vaginal itching, irritation, and a watery discharge. Often the vaginal epithelium and cervical epithelium are quite inflamed. Protozoa live in the secretions and can be seen under the microscope when they are placed in a drop of saline. They move because they possess a tail or flagellum, and the diagnosis is made when such an organism about the size of a white blood cell is seen moving rapidly across the slide.

While some relief may be obtained from the antiyeast imidazole medications, the specific therapy is metronidazole, an antibiotic that is effective against this organism. Metronidazole can be given in one dose of 2 grams or two doses of 1 gram each separated by twelve hours, or it can be taken from five to seven days, 500 mg three times a day. For persistent or recurrent cases, metronidazole may be given 500 mg, three times a day for fourteen days. The partner of a sexually active woman is likely to be infected and should be treated at the same time she is treated.

Often when a trichamonas infection is treated with metronidazole, the organisms are rapidly killed. If yeast is present in the vagina, there will be a flare-up of the yeast infection. Therefore, it is frequently useful to use a vaginal antiyeast cream at the same time a patient is being treated for trichamonas.

Bacterial Vaginosis

This is a condition in which multiple types of bacteria overgrow the vagina so that not only is there an increase in numbers of types of bacteria, but there are also increased numbers of the bacteria themselves. The reason for this is unknown. The condition is quite common in young women but also occurs in older women. The diagnosis is made because of a watery discharge with a foul odor. The diagnosis is also helped by finding multiple bacteria fixed to the surface of epithelial cells when a sample of the cells is taken with a cotton applicator from the wall of the vagina and placed in a drop of saline. The cells are called clue cells and are diagnostic for bacterial vaginosis. The treatment is 2 grams of metronidazole in a single dose, but it may also be treated effectively with vaginal clindomycin cream, one applicator at bedtime for seven nights, or metronidazole gel one to two applicators per day for five to seven days. A variety of other antibiotics can be given, but they are no more effective than are metronidazole or clindomycin. Women with susceptibility to bacterial vaginosis frequently have recurrences.

OTHER PROBLEMS

Older women are susceptible to other diseases that may involve the vagina and vulva. One of these is the herpes virus, which can attack as a primary infection in women who come in contact with it, or it can occur as a recurrence of previous herpes infections. Generally, a primary infection will last about two weeks and will have both local and general effects. The local effect will be the production of vesicles and ulcers on the vulva, in the vagina, and on the cervix. These may be associated with a severe inflammation causing edema of the vulva, pain, and difficulty in urinating. General (systemic) symptoms include stiff neck and headache because of irritation of the covering of the brain (the meninges), irritation of the liver causing abdominal pain, and severe flulike symptoms of muscle aches and pains, fever, and just plain feeling bad. The disease will frequently be self-limited, and the severe symptoms will disappear in about two weeks, but the length and severity may be modified with the drug acyclovir. This can be given in 200 mg doses five times a day or by IV use. Certainly, anyone with a primary herpetic infection should consult a physician and be evaluated and properly treated.

Recurrent herpes infections are fairly common but vary from woman to woman. Generally they cause lesser degrees of symptoms, most often local vesicles and ulcers on the vulva, and the attacks generally last three to five days. Women who are prone to frequent recurrences can use acyclovir in a chronic fashion.

Another viral condition that can occur in older women just as in younger women is infection with human papilloma virus (HPV, wart virus). While the development of warts on the vulva or vagina can be annoying, they can be destroyed by local therapy. Unfortunately, the virus remains in the body forever, and some women are prone to recurrences. There is an epidemiologic relationship between vulvar cancer and the wart virus in younger women, but this same relationship has not been seen in vulvar disease in older women. This may be because this viral condition is not as common in women who are currently in the older age group. This relationship may change as infected younger woman age. There is also an epidemiologic relationship between HPV and cervical cancer, but a cause-and-effect relationship has not been shown. Therapy for the development of warts on the perineum is local destruction. There are no antiviral agents for HPV infection currently available.

Conclusions

The vulva and vagina are prone to develop several different conditions in older women. Some are potentially serious. It is always prudent to consult a physician for any condition that does not rapidly clear up with the use of the usual over-the-counter medications. Lesions that linger should be evaluated and in most cases biopsied. Do not ignore chronic problems in this area of your body.

CHAPTER 14

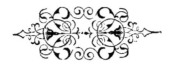

Urinary Incontinence and Other
Bladder Problems

Urinary incontinence is a common problem in the elderly. Ten to 15 percent of older women living in their homes in the community have varying degrees of incontinence. One study demonstrated that 40 percent of women over the age of seventy who are hospitalized, are incontinent. Other studies have shown that between 40 and 60 percent of women in nursing homes are incontinent. While the problem has major social and medical implications, it causes such embarrassment to the sufferers that it may lead to their limiting their social contacts, activities outside the home, and, in some cases, employment opportunities. What is even worse is that their embarrassment may be such that they do not bring it to the attention of their physicians. Continence is a complicated issue that involves an interaction of the patient's neurologic state, mental status, and anatomical and hormonal balance. It also can be greatly influenced by medications that the patient may be taking.

This chapter discusses continence and the loss of continence from many facets, explaining the reasons for the loss of urinary control and the steps that can be taken to restore control. The chapter also describes other diseases and conditions of the bladder that may affect older women.

CONTINENCE

Continence is a function of the ability of the urethra to prevent the flow of urine and the ability of the bladder to store urine. The urethra is the tube that drains the bladder. Voiding is dependent upon the ability of the urethra to relax and the muscles of the bladder to contract. Both the urethra and the bladder are under the control of the autonomic nervous system and specifically the part of the nervous system which is referred to as the autonomic nervous system. This portion of the nervous system is responsible for many bodily functions such as control of heart rate, blood pressure, breathing, digestion, and bladder function. The autonomic nervous system is divided into two portions; the sympathetic system, which is under the control of the neurotransmitter norepinephrine, and the parasympathetic system, which is under the control of the neurotransmitter acetyl choline. These neurotransmitters regulate all of the body functions described above and medications are frequently designed to stimulate or block the actions of the neurotransmitters norepinephrine and acetyl chlorine in order to relieve symptoms involving the various bodily functions. If a medication is being given to reduce blood pressure, it may block the neurotransmitter responsible for increasing blood pressure, but it may also inadvertently interfere with other bodily functions that utilize that required neurotransmitter.

Interestingly, the neurotransmitters work through receptor sites in the various organs that they serve. The sympathetic nervous system neurotransmitter norepinephrine works on sites known as alpha- and beta-receptors. Alpha-receptors are abundant in the bladder neck and urethra but absent in the bladder. When they are stimulated they cause contraction of the muscles that they serve. Therefore, stimulating the sympathetic nervous system and increasing the amount of norepinephrine causes contraction of the bladder neck and urethra and aids continence. Since there are no alpha-receptors in the bladder, the bladder remains relaxed, which is what it must do to store urine. Furthermore, when norepinephrine stimulates beta-receptors, the result is a relaxation of the muscles involved. The bladder wall is rich in beta-receptors, but the urethra has none. The sympathetic nervous system's responsibility in continence is to cause contraction of the urethra and relaxation of the bladder, thereby preventing the urine from passing and allowing it to be stored.

Through its neurotransmitter, acetyl choline, the parasympathetic nervous system is responsible for voiding. It causes contraction of the bladder muscle and relaxation of the urethra. Thus, continence is a balance between the activities of the sympathetic and the parasympathetic nervous systems. Clearly, medications that affect either one of these can affect continence, either by causing difficulty in voiding, sometimes known as hesitancy, or by causing dribbling or outright loss of urine.

Neurologically the problem is even more complex. Clearly, the brain and the spinal cord need to be involved in the voiding process or the whole reflex would be automatic, and whenever the bladder filled with urine it would empty. Since this would be inconvenient for most people, control by the brain must be superimposed. The brain's role is twofold; first, to prevent the emptying of the bladder at inconvenient times by sending a signal to interrupt the bladder-emptying reflex, and second, to send a signal to allow the bladder to empty when it is convenient. These signals are sent through the spinal cord to the micturation center, which controls the actual emptying of the bladder and is low in the spinal cord. The long nerves that run from the brain to the micturation center can be interfered with by vascular disease or by tumors of the brain or spinal cord. They also can be damaged by such illnesses as Parkinson's disease, multiple sclerosis, diabetic neuropathy (the late stage of diabetes mellitus), and a host of other conditions. Also, medications of various sorts can interfere with the function of the nerves. Irritation of the bladder caused by infection, tumors, or irradiation may increase the stimulation coming from the bladder to the nervous system to such an extent that it overcomes the central nervous system's ability to control the bladder.

It is clear that medications play an important role in control of continence. Table 14.1 lists a group of commonly used medications, the reasons they are used, and their action on bladder function.

Anatomical relationships of the urethra and bladder are also important in maintaining continence. The strength of the muscles that contract the urethra and bladder neck is important, as are the relationships of the urethra and the bladder within the abdominal cavity and pelvis. The urethra itself has both smooth and striated muscles. These are at their strongest when a woman is in her late teens and early twenties and tend to become weaker with time. It is possible to measure the pressure within the urethra that is the result of both the strength of the urethral muscles and the elasticity of the urethral wall. The muscles of the urethra and the elasticity of the wall are supported by estrogen. Therefore, after menopause these structures weaken rapidly, and the pressure within the urethra goes down. One form of incontinence related to low pressure within the urethra is seen primarily in women past the age of fifty. There is also a plexus of veins surrounding the bladder neck that is also under the influence of estrogen and is most predominant when a woman is younger. The pressure of the blood within this plexus of vessels is directly related to the pressure created by the heartbeat and contributes to maintaining the urethral closing pressure. As this plexus weakens, this extra bit of protection is partially lost. Finally, the muscles of the pelvis that constrict the ure-

TABLE 14.1.   Medications That Can Interfere With Bladder Function

Drug	Usual Indication	Action
Reserpine	Hypertension	Incontinence
Methyldopa	Hypertension	Incontinence
Bromocriptine (Parlodel)	To treat breast secretions	Causes bladder neck obstruction (hesitancy)
Levodopa	Parkinson's disease	Bladder neck obstruction; difficulty voiding
Digitalis	Heart disease	Decreased bladder capacity by increasing bladder wall tension
Major tranquilizers (Thorazine, Compazine, Haloperidol, and others)	Treat many psychiatric conditions	Incontinence
Isoxsuprine	Dilate blood vessels	Urinary retention by inhibiting bladder muscle contraction
Terbutaline	Bronchodilator (asthma)	Urinary retention (inhibits bladder muscle contraction)
Caffeine	Stimulant	Incontinence: dribbling

thra are important in contributing to the urethral closing pressure. Studies have shown that these vessels have their greatest effect in the middle 60 percent of the urethral length. These are the muscles that are strengthened with isometric Kegel exercises.

The anatomical relationship of the urethra, bladder neck, and bladder are also very important in maintaining continence. Normally, the bladder neck, upper urethra, and bladder are all present within the abdominal cavity. Therefore, an increase in intra-abdominal pressure, such as the pressure that occurs with a cough or sneeze or straining, is brought to bear equally on the bladder, bladder neck, and upper urethra. However, if the pelvic support structure is weakened and the bladder neck and urethra are allowed to slip into the pelvis and out of the abdominal cavity, then an increase in intra-abdominal pressure is added to the pressure within the bladder and is usually enough to overcome urethral closing pressure, thereby causing incontinence, usually seen in the form of a spurt of urine. This type of incontinence is referred to as genuine stress incontinence.

Multiple factors affect continence, including the neurologic status of the patient, the anatomical relationships of the bladder neck and urethra, and the health of the bladder and urethra. These functions are clearly affected by outside forces such as medications or illnesses, and it is the job of the physician to sort these out, to decide the reason for the patient's problem, and to find a therapy that will work in the individual case.

Evaluation of Incontinence

If you suffer from incontinence and bring it to the attention of your physician, your evaluation should begin with your physician's taking a detailed medical, urologic, and neurologic history in order to identify all of the possible contributing factors. The medical history is important to identify conditions that may be contributing to your incontinence and also to detect medications you may be taking for other purposes that may be affecting your ability to control your urine.

A urologic history should include information regarding how long you have been incontinent and under what circumstances you lose urine. In other words, do you lose urine when you cough or sneeze or while climbing stairs? Do you have a feeling of urgency; do you need to get up during the night to go to the bathroom, and if so, how many times? Do you have to void frequently, or can you hold your urine for long periods of time? Do you dribble? Do you have difficulty starting your voiding stream, do you take long periods of time to empty your bladder, or do you have painful urination? Has there been blood or pus in your urine?

Your physician will also want to know whether or not you are taking hormone replacement therapy and, of course, whether or not you have had any procedures or treatments that could affect your pelvic organs or your urinary tract.

Another important factor that your doctor will want to know about is whether or not you have incontinence of stool. In many situations, when the patient suffers from neurologic disease, incontinence of stool is also present, indicating a general pelvic floor dysfunction. On the other hand, chronic constipation and stool impaction may contribute but for other reasons such as poor diet, poor fluid intake, overuse of cathartics, and so on.

The doctor will then do a physical examination to detect evidence for anatomic or neurologic disease involving the pelvic floor.

There are several tests that may be utilized to help make a diagnosis. Unfortunately, most of the simple tests that can be done in the office are not totally diagnostic but can contribute to the doctor's clinical impression, which of course will be helped by the history and physical examination. The gold standard today for determining the type of incontinence you may have is urodynamic studies. These are generally carried out using machines that allow for the simultaneous measurement of intra-abdominal pressure and the pressure within the urethra and the bladder. The data that are obtained will allow the physician to determine the type of incontinence you may have. There are, however, several tests that can be run simply in the office to help the physician make a diagnosis. These are most useful for women who have never been treated for their incontinence. The way they may be done is as follows: You are asked to void, and the amount of urine that you void is measured. The doctor then places a catheter into your bladder and measures the amount of urine left in the bladder after voiding (residual urine). This should be less than 50 ml. If it is more, this may imply that you have a cystocele, a bulging of your bladder into the vagina, which becomes a place for urine to be collected and not voided, or it may mean that you are not emptying your bladder properly for a number of other reasons. The physician will then instill warm saline, salt water, into your bladder to determine when you have your first urge to void and when you have a strong urge to void. This will give the physician some idea of the irritability of your bladder and of your bladder capacity. Most women will have their first urge to void when 200 to 250 ml of saline have been instilled in their bladder, and by 400 to 500 ml they will have a strong urge to void. This implies normal bladder capacity and function. If the first urge to void occurs at 50 to 100 ml of saline and a very strong urge is present by 200 to 250 ml, you probably have an irritable bladder or a bladder of small capacity. If, on the other hand, you do not note an urge to void as the bladder is filled to large capacity, you may have a neurologic bladder. This is a condition in which the normal nerve messages are not getting through to the brain and the bladder is just being allowed to fill without any knowledge on your part. This is frequently seen in the conditions that affect the nerves running from the spinal cord to the brain, in such conditions as multiple sclerosis or diabetic neuropathy, and in other neurologic diseases.

When the doctor has made these determinations, it is possible to remove the saline, leaving 250 ml within the bladder. The doctor can then ask you to cough, and if you lose urine in a spurt it may indicate genuine stress incontinence. The bladder neck can then be supported and the process repeated. If this prevents the spurt, that is some evidence that the problem may indeed be genuine stress incontinence. This test is not always accurate, and there are several ways in which the results can be misleading, but it does give the physician an idea of the type of incontinence you may have.

Some physicians have instruments in their office for measuring pressure within the urethra and the bladder. This allows them to get an idea of whether or not your problem is genuine stress incontinence or a form of urgency incontinence, sometimes

TABLE 14.2.   Symptoms in Stress and Urgency Incontinence

Symptoms	Stress	Urgency
Frequency	–	++
Urgency	–	++
Getting up at night to urinate	–	++
Amount of urine lost with cough	Small	Large

known as bladder dysfunction. It is important to make this differentiation, as it has been shown in many large studies that about one third of the patients have both components, and treatment will only be successful if both are treated. If a diagnosis of genuine stress incontinence is made and an operation performed, if the patient has a bladder dysfunction component, she may still not be continent after the operation. This, of course, can be very frustrating for the patient as well as for the doctor.

If, on the basis of your history, physical examination, and simple office testing, a diagnosis can clearly be made, your doctor may institute therapy without going to the more expensive urodynamic studies. If, however, you have had previous incontinence surgery or if your case is unclear after the office procedures, urodynamic studies should be ordered.

Table 14.2 demonstrates the differences between genuine stress incontinence and bladder dysfunction-urge incontinence. Again, these represent guidelines for the physician, but in most patients there is overlap of symptomatology making it difficult to make a diagnosis only on the basis of the history.

TREATMENT OF INCONTINENCE

The treatment of incontinence depends upon the type of incontinence. Studies have shown that roughly 40 to 45 percent of newly diagnosed incontinent women suffer from genuine stress incontinence, 20 to 25 percent from urgency incontinence, and the rest from a mixture of the two, thus making the proper diagnosis before starting treatment important. The treatment of genuine stress incontinence can be nonsurgical, but often it is necessary to perform an operative procedure to cure the condition.

The nonsurgical therapy of genuine stress incontinence consists of placing the patient on hormone replacement therapy if possible. This will improve bladder and urethral function by improving the elasticity and muscle strength of the urethra and bladder neck as well as improving the vascularity of the organs themselves. In addition, estrogen stimulates the production of alpha-receptors, which are important to allow the urethra to contract. Perhaps the most important function of estrogen is to produce collagen, which is the component of connective tissue that strengthens the pelvic support structures. It is not uncommon to see women with poor pelvic support structures improve on estrogen alone and to see the incontinence disappear.

Along with estrogen therapy, pelvic exercises to strengthen the muscles that surround the urethra and vagina are equally important. In the 1950s, A.H. Kegel designed isometric exercises aimed at these pelvic muscles. Originally he suggested that contraction of these muscles be done ten to twenty times starting with arising in the morning and continuing every half hour throughout the day. Needless to say, this took a great deal of effort, and most women did not care to make it. Later, Kegel showed that modifying this regimen to performing these exercises three to four times a day would work equally well. Learning to contract the proper muscles is the key to success of these exercises. In the physician's office, during a pelvic examination, the physician may demonstrate which muscles need to be contracted. Another way a woman can learn to contract the proper muscles is to consider trying to stop her urinary stream while urinating. The muscles that are contracted to accomplish this are the muscles that must be contracted during the Kegel exercises.

A variety of other means have been devised to strengthen these muscles. Most of the work came from England, where there are long periods of waiting for surgical procedures to be performed due to the changes in the medical care brought about by the National Health Plan in Great Britain. In order to try to alleviate symptoms of incontinence in women waiting for surgical procedures, many variations on the Kegel exercises were developed. One utilizes weighted plastic cones, which a woman is instructed to carry within her vagina. In order to keep the cones from falling out, the muscles must be contracted. As the muscles strengthen, heavier cones can be accommodated. This variation on the Kegel exercises is an effective one but probably no more effective than the isometric exercises designed by Kegel.

Another approach utilizes biofeedback. It is possible to put into the vagina an appliance attached to a transducer that can be hooked up to a television screen. It is then possible to visualize the strength of contractions of the vaginal constrictor muscles by seeing the strength of the contraction depicted as a graph on the screen. This allows the woman to have some idea of how hard she needs to contract the muscles, and over time she can build the strength of these muscles, essentially before her very eyes. While this technique has become quite popular in Britain, it has not yet caught on in the United States. With the use of estrogens and pelvic exercises, cures of 30 to 70 percent have been reported in various studies.

A number of surgical procedures have been designed to address the problem of genuine stress incontinence. It is difficult to say which procedure is best, because often this depends upon the problem that the specific woman has, as well as the experience of the surgeon with a specific procedure. Comparing the results of various procedures from one clinic to another can be misleading. Since the problem is usually anatomical, that is, the displacement of the bladder neck and upper urethra to a lower position in the pelvis, most surgical procedures are designed to correct this. The choices of procedures include a vaginal approach, an abdominal approach, or a combination of the two.

The vaginal approach is useful if there is obvious prolapse of the pelvic organs.

Such prolapse involves a cystocele, which is the bulging of the bladder into the anterior wall of the vagina; a rectocele, which is a bulging of the rectum into the posterior wall of the vagina; a prolapse of the uterus, which is a descent of the cervix and uterus through the vaginal canal; or an enterocele, which is a hernia of the abdominal cavity through the posterior wall of the vagina. If such a pelvic organ prolapse is present, surgery that includes a vaginal approach is appropriate in order to restore anatomical relationships. The vaginal procedure performed for a cystocele repair is called an anterior colporrhaphy. The problem is generally that the fascial covering between the vagina and the bladder, known as the pubocervical fascia, is stretched and splayed out. This occurs because of childbirth or other pelvic trauma. The cystocele repair involves isolating this fascia and restoring its integrity. Sutures are generally placed at the bladder neck as well both to plicate the lower urethra and to help support the bladder neck behind the pubic symphysis.

It is an interesting embryologic and anatomical observation that the muscular sphincter around the upper urethra is not donut-shaped but rather is shaped like a horseshoe. With time, stress, and relaxation of the muscles of this area, the upper urethra stretches, and a funneling effect takes place. The plication sutures placed at the bladder neck can partially overcome this.

Other vaginal operations that have been designed to be used as part of this procedure have as their purpose the replacement of the bladder neck behind the pubic symphysis. These procedures utilize special needles to place suture around the bladder neck, suspending it to structures in the anterior abdominal wall, primarily the fascia covering the abdominal wall muscles. The best known of these procedures are the Pereyra procedure and the Stamey modification of this procedure. These procedures have been met with various success but are certainly not 100 percent effective.

Procedures performed through an abdominal incision attempt to reestablish the relationship of the bladder neck behind the pubic symphysis. A number of such procedures have been devised, and they are often quite effective. The best known of these are the Burch procedure and the Marshall Marchetti Krantz procedure. Each uses different structures to which the bladder neck area is fixed, and each has its supporters. Both are useful, and I generally use the one that fits the patient's anatomical needs the best.

Occasionally the defect in the pubocervical fascia is not central but rather lateral; the pubocervical fascia is torn from its attachments to other pelvic structures laterally rather than being damaged centrally, as is usually the case. In such situations, a good result can be obtained by performing a paravaginal repair. This procedure is also performed through an abdominal incision.

A variety of other operations have been developed. One group, sling procedures, have a specific application in women whose genuine stress incontinence is due to a low pressure in the urethra.

Clearly, there are a number of procedures which can be applied to solve this surgical problem. The best choice should depend upon the specific anatomical problem that the individual patient demonstrates. If the procedure is carefully chosen to fit the patient's needs, success rates in the neighborhood of 90 percent can be anticipated.

However, women who require these procedures generally have anatomical weakness, and recurrences will often occur with time.

Women with genuine stress incontinence due to an anatomical displacement of the bladder neck usually have hypermobility of the bladder neck and upper urethra. There is, however, a form of genuine stress incontinence that does not have hypermobility of the bladder neck; rather the incontinence is due to a low pressure within the urethra and a tendency to funnel at the bladder neck. This is seen in older women because of changes in the musculature and elastic fibers of the urethra due to the lack of estrogen and to the general aging process, but it is also seen in women who have had multiple operations and whose urethras have become stiffened and less able to contract. Often known as stovepipe urethras, these are seen in both women who have had multiple surgical procedures and in women who have had irradiation for pelvic neoplasm. This form of incontinence is known as intrinsic sphincter deficiency (ISD). There are basically three ways of managing this at the present time.

The first is to perform a sling procedure, which implies the placement of either a piece of the woman's own fascia or an inert material such as mersilene beneath the urethra, fixing it to the anterior abdominal wall. Thus, when the woman coughs or sneezes, the abdominal wall muscles contract, pulling up on the sling and stopping the loss of urine. The second therapy involves the placement of an artificial bladder sphincter. This is essentially a cuff that goes around the bladder neck and can be filled with mercury from a reservoir, the control of which can be placed in the labia. The woman can empty the mercury from the cuff and allow the urine to flow when she wishes to void and then refill the cuff when she wishes to be continent. Each of these methods has its advocates. The sling procedures are close to 100 percent effective in this condition but have the disadvantage that some women do not void spontaneously for quite some time, necessitating self-catheterization. The problem with the artificial sphincter is that since it is inert material, it sometimes sloughs out of the woman's body.

More recently, bovine collagen injections into the periurethral space have been utilized for ISD. For the appropriate woman, this is quite effective therapy. It can be carried out as an outpatient procedure, with the injections being performed through a urethrascope, and effectively the procedure allows for a bulking up of the funneling of the bladder neck, thereby closing down the diameter of the upper urethra. To date, success has been reported for between 80 and 90 percent of these women. The only drawback has been that many women prove to be allergic to bovine collagen. Women should be skin tested for this allergy prior to injection. The material is fairly expensive, but because the procedure can be done on an outpatient basis, it is less expensive than the other two alternatives. Only time will tell whether or not injections will need to be repeated. Since bovine collagen is an organic substance, it is possible that the body will eventually break it down, requiring repeat injection. On the other hand, it may cause enough scarring during the healing process that the desired results may be obtained without further injection. Not all medical centers are able to perform this procedure, but training programs are available and it is becoming more and more available throughout the country.

CASE STUDY

Myra is a sixty-two-year-old woman who has undergone several procedures for incontinence in the past. Although she has taken estrogen replacement therapy from time to time, she has not taken it for the past five years because of the fear that it may cause breast cancer. Her two sisters have had breast cancer, and she is very concerned about this possibility. For the past year and a half she has noticed increased loss of urine when she coughs, sneezes, runs up and down stairs, or lifts a heavy object.

Her pelvic examination did not reveal a major anatomical defect, but on uro-dynamic study she was found to have a stress urinary incontinence problem and a low pressure in her urethra. She was diagnosed with intrinsic urethral sphincter dysfunction, and the three means of therapy were discussed with her. She elected to try bovine collagen injection, and after being successfully skin tested without any evidence of allergy, she underwent an injection of 10 ml of material on either side of her urethra. The physician doing the procedure noted a funneling of the urethra prior to the beginning of the procedure and good closure of the urethra after the procedure was completed. One year after completing the injection, Myra is still continent.

BLADDER INSTABILITY-URGE INCONTINENCE

This essentially is the involuntary uninhibited contraction of the bladder during the storage phase. The International Continence Society has renamed what were called bladder instabilities to designate a group of conditions related to the primary cause. Be that as it may, from the standpoint of the patient, loss of urine is usually involuntary, related to urge, frequency, and, at times, discomfort during urination. It is the physician's responsibility to try to pinpoint the reason for the bladder dysfunction, and if it is due to something that can be eliminated, such as a bladder infection, then this should be the first step in its management. Often the dysfunction is not related to something that can be identified and appropriately treated. Therefore, management is aimed at quieting the bladder. If the problem is a pattern of frequent urination, it may be useful to retrain the bladder to maintain larger capacities.

The woman who feels a need to void often and voids small amounts can slowly prolong the interval between bathroom stops to retrain her bladder to increase the volume it can comfortably contain. This approach has been studied in several medical centers and is known to be effective, providing there is no pathology in the bladder itself.

Since the bladder contractions are mediated through the parasympathetic nervous system via the neurotransmitter acetyl choline, most medications that counteract undesirable bladder activity are cholinergic, that is, agents that interfere with this function. The oldest such medication is atropine, which relaxes the bladder quite well but often has undesirable side effects, most commonly dry mouth. A group of other medications are equally useful but with fewer side effects. Examples of these are propantheline (Pro-Banthine) in doses of 15 to 30 mg four times a day; flavoxate

(Urispas) in doses of 200 mg every six hours, and oxybutynin chloride (Ditropan) 5 mg every eight to twelve hours. All of these agents are antispasmodic, anticholenergic drugs. One side effect that must be guarded against is that they can cause acute glaucoma attacks in women with glaucoma. This is a condition that involves increased intraocular pressure and is moderately common in older individuals. Therefore, before starting such medications, women should have an eye examination to measure intraocular pressures.

Other agents that have similar effects are tricyclic antidepressants such as imipramine. These can be given in very low doses, usually at bedtime, and will relax the bladder sufficiently so that most women will get a good night's sleep. The antidepressant effect probably also contributes to their usefulness.

Other medications that may be available in the future belong to the group of calcium channel blockers. This is a common group of medications for treating high blood pressure. The specific agent of this family that has a unique effect on the bladder is not yet available in the United States. As with other types of incontinence, estrogen therapy is often of value.

CASE STUDY

Josie is a seventy-two-year-old thin female who has been widowed for five years. From the time she was a little girl she has urinated frequently. In the beginning she did not have to get up during the night to urinate, but would urinate at least every hour to two hours during the day, at least in small amounts. She denies any discomfort and states that she has needed to urinate frequently for as long as she can remember.

She went through menopause at age fifty-one and has not used estrogen replacement therapy. For the past fifteen years she has been getting up at least once a night and more recently, two and three times during the night. In the morning, she needs to rush to the bathroom to keep from losing urine. Throughout the day, she voids every twenty minutes to one hour, relatively small amounts of urine. She does not have any pain, backache, chills, or fever.

On urodynamic study, she was found to have a first urge to void when 75 ml of saline was placed in her bladder and a strong urge to void when 150 ml of saline was present in her bladder. Otherwise, the exam of her urethra and bladder were completely normal. Urine sent for culture at the start of the urodynamic procedure was sterile for bacteria, and it was determined she had urgency incontinence.

Josie was started on a course of bladder training in which she increased the time between voiding by ten minutes for the first several days, increasing by twenty minutes and then thirty minutes, and finally over time to a point where she could avoid urinating for three hours at a time. During that time she was treated with Pro-Banthine 15 mg four times a day. She was also started on estrogen replacement therapy. On this regimen she has done very well, and after six months she is able to go three to four hours between voids and gets up only once during each night.

This is a typical history of a woman who has needed to empty her bladder frequently throughout her life. As she has gotten older, two changes related to the aging process have made matters worse. The first is the tendency for the kidneys to no longer concentrate urine so that she could get through the night without filling her bladder. The second is the fact that without estrogen therapy, the epithelium of the bladder becomes much thinner and the bladder itself more irritable. The estrogen helped improve her bladder health, and the Pro-Banthine and bladder retraining improved bladder capacity and decreased the urge to void. Because her kidneys still do not concentrate as well as they did when she was younger, she still finds it necessary to get up once a night to urinate.

OTHER TYPES OF INCONTINENCE

There are other types of incontinence. The first is true incontinence, which involves a fistulous tract between the ureter, bladder, or urethra and the vagina. This condition generally follows an obstetrical or surgical injury or irradiation therapy for cancer. The incontinence is continuous, as the urine passes through the opening into the vagina as it is excreted into the bladder. Therapy for this is surgical repair.

Overflow incontinence is a condition that is associated with neurologic disease, including multiple sclerosis, Parkinson's disease, diabetic neuropathy, trauma, and tumors of the central nervous system. It is best treated by dealing, if possible, with the causative condition. Most patients with this problem need to learn the technique of self-catheterization, because no medications are known that are capable of treating this condition.

BLADDER INFECTIONS

Lower urinary tract infections are common in women of all ages and especially in older women. It has been estimated that as many as 25 percent of women in the United States experience an episode of acute urinary tract infection annually. Symptoms include frequency, urgency, painful urination, and possibly blood in the urine (hematuria) or pus in the urine (pyuria). In addition, the women may complain of backache, pain in the pelvis or flank, chills, and fever. With infection, there may be dribbling or incontinence. Ninety percent of acute cystitis is due to infection with two bacteria, Escherichia coli and staphylococcus. However, a variety of other organisms may be found. When women complain of such symptoms, a urinalysis may reveal bacteria, white blood cells, and red blood cells. A culture should always be taken to identify the specific infectious agent. Urine for culture is generally obtained by performing a clean voided sample. This involves the washing of the perineum with a soap solution and catching the stream while separating the labia. In this way, vaginal discharge to the container can be avoided. Since vaginal discharge almost always contains bacteria, this would confuse the culture picture. After a culture is obtained, it is appropriate to treat the woman with a broad spectrum antibiotic or sulfa preparation and to await the culture results. Generally, within forty-eight hours the culture report is back, and if the agent being used is not specific for the organism, the antibiotic may be changed.

It has been estimated that roughly 10 percent of women over the age of seventy who are otherwise healthy have positive urine cultures even though they are asymptomatic. Between ages seventy and eighty this figure increases to about 20 percent, and up to 80 percent of women over age eighty will have bacteria in their urine without symptoms. It is difficult to prove whether or not this is of clinical significance. In general, if bacteria are found in the urine of asymptomatic women, most physicians will treat. Screening older populations for the presence of asymptomatic infection has not been proven to be of value, since no long-term problem has been found in such women.

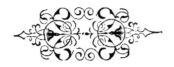

CHAPTER 15

Pelvic Support Problems

Pelvic support structures frequently weaken as women age. Some women have support weaknesses from birth that become more accentuated over time. In other women, the support structures of the pelvis are weakened by childbirth, physical injury, or damage sustained from chronic straining, by nerve damage, or, in some cases, because of multiple surgical procedures. In addition, lack of estrogen, seen in many postmenopausal women who do not take estrogen replacement therapy, causes a weakening of the pelvic support tissue and their blood supply. This chapter describes the types of pelvic support problems, their consequences, and the way they may be treated.

ANATOMICAL CONSIDERATIONS

Several structures and groups of structures are responsible for the support of the pelvic organs. The most important of these is the pelvic diaphragm. This is composed of two strong muscles, the coccygeus and levator ani muscles with their fascia covering, which form a sling for the pelvic organs. Interestingly, these muscles evolved from the tail-wagging musculature of four-legged animals. They are very strong, with interwoven bundles of muscle fibers that completely close off the pelvis except for openings for the urethra, vagina, and rectum, which they encircle. The levator ani muscle is the largest and strongest and is really composed of three major components. The total muscles mass extends from the pubic symphysis at the front of the pelvic to the coccyx (tailbone) at the back of the pelvis and is fixed to the lateral walls on each side. The coccygeus reinforces the posterior portion of the pelvic diaphragm. The levator ani muscles play a major role in controlling urination, maintaining fecal continence, and supporting the organs of the abdominal cavity and pelvis. They also play an important role in the birth process, helping in the expulsion of the fetus.

There is a second musculofascial diaphragm, called the urogenital diaphragm, which contributes to pelvic support and is closer to the outer portion of the perineum. It supports the anterior portion of the pelvic outlet and consists of three separate muscles, the ischeocavernosus, bulbocavernosus, and transverse perineal muscles. These are all in front of the rectum but do support the vagina and the front part of the woman's perineum. They also contribute to urinary continence. Both diaphragms are rich in blood vessels and nerves. For the most part, the nerves that transverse them are important for the innervation of the pelvic floor. Damage to these nerves can lead to loss of sensation or loss of strength in the muscles of the pelvic diaphragm, and it may decrease the strength of the pelvic supports.

There are other supporting ligaments for the pelvic organs. While they are called ligaments, they are really thickenings of the fascia that surround various muscles and other structures. The vagina and cervix are surrounded by the endopelvic fascia, which is primarily present between the vagina and cervix and the bladder anteriorly. The cervix is supported by the cardinal ligaments laterally and the uterosacral ligaments posteriorly, which blend themselves into the endopelvic fascia. Unfortunately, there is no fascial covering between the rectum and the vagina posteriorly. The support here is often the responsibility of the levator ani muscles.

The uterosacral ligaments and cardinal ligaments are very important in preventing the cervix and uterus from prolapsing through the vaginal tube. The endopelvic fascia that is between the bladder and the vagina is the important support of the bladder, preventing a bulge of the bladder into the vagina (cystocele). If the rectum bulges into the vagina, it is called a rectocele. Good supports by the uterosacral ligaments help to protect the floor of the abdominal cavity and prevent the development of a hernia into the posterior wall of the vagina (enterocele).

All of these structures are important in maintaining the strength of the pelvic supports and preventing pelvic relaxation problems. Undue pressure upon them, such as is seen in very obese women, trauma most often associated with childbirth, and other factors such as hormone withdrawal or nerve damage will detract from the strength of the pelvic supports.

THE ROLE OF ESTROGEN

Estrogen is responsible for the health and integrity of the epithelial lining of the bladder and the vagina, for the blood supply to the pelvic structures, and for the strength and thickness of the fascia and ligaments. The bulk of the tissue making up fascia and ligaments is collagen, whose development is stimulated by estrogen. Therefore, estrogen plays a major role in tissue supports. In treating women with pelvic relaxation problems, I always begin them on estrogen first, providing there is no contraindication. Although estrogen cannot be expected to correct all pelvic anatomical problems, it is surprising how often improvement occurs. Occasionally I have seen total prolapses of the uterus through the introitus regress with the return to near normal anatomically on estrogen therapy alone. Surprisingly, this can happen in two to three months. Even if regression of the anatomical defect does not take place on estrogen, the improvement of the quality of the tissue and its blood supply makes for a greater chance of success with surgical procedures. Therefore, all women with pelvic support problems who can take estrogen should do so.

PELVIC SUPPORT DISORDERS

If weakening of the pelvic support structures occurs, the resultant problem may be a prolapse of the urethra (urethrocele), the bladder neck, the bladder (cystocele), and the rectum (rectocele) into the vaginal tube. It may also lead to the development of a hernia from the posterior aspect of the floor of the abdominal cavity into the area of the posterior vagina (enterocele) or prolapse of the uterus and cervix down the vagina and perhaps out of the vaginal opening (descensus). Often a variety of these conditions occur in the same woman.

Urethrocele and Cystocele

A weakening of or damage to the endopelvic fascia may lead to the prolapse of the urethra and bladder neck (urethrocele) and the bladder (cystocele) into the anterior wall of the vagina. The bulge may be contained within the vagina itself or may actually protrude through the opening of the vagina. If the urethra and the bladder neck are part of the bulge, the woman is generally incontinent of urine. If only the bladder is part of the bulge and the urethra and bladder neck remain suspended in their normal position, she may not be incontinent of urine but may have a large urine residual after voiding. This may lead to a feeling of inability to empty the bladder completely, and because there is stasis of urine within the bladder, a bladder infection may occur. Thus, the symptoms the woman notes may be stress urinary incontinence, a feeling of urgency; a sensation of incomplete emptying after voiding; and a feeling that structures may be falling out of the vagina. If the cystocele protrudes through the vagina, the woman may be aware of a small bulging mass, and at times she may need to replace this into the vagina in order to void. The mass, if present, will generally get larger with straining. After time, it may remain outside the introitus all of the time.

The physician notes the cystocele when examining the woman in stirrups but will probably want to examine her standing as well to note the full effect of the bulge. By identifying the location of the bladder neck, the physician will also be able to tell whether or not the bulge includes a urethrocele and a prolapse of the bladder neck. If a urethrocele is present, the woman is usually incontinent to some degree, and the physician may note a urine odor about the perineum.

Urethroceles and cystoceles are almost always found in women who have had children. They have been noted in women who have never been pregnant but who have poor structural support. This is sometimes seen because of congenital malformations of the abdominal wall and pelvis or weakness of the musculature and connective tissue of the pelvic floor secondary to chronic straining, trauma, or other forces. All pelvic structure weaknesses are made worse by coughing, so smokers and people with chronic lung disease are more prone to develop these.

Not all cystoceles are symptomatic, and those that do not bulge from the vagina may not need any therapy. I have followed women for years who have had moderate-sized cystoceles but no symptoms associated with them and have not noted that they get any worse. On the other hand, this is unpredictable, and women with pelvic relaxation problems usually do get progressive changes.

Specific therapy for cystoceles and urethroceles can be nonsurgical or surgical. Certainly the woman is entitled to a trial of estrogen therapy and pelvic exercises. This should always be tried for several month before resorting to surgery, as many improve surprisingly. There are a variety of appliances called pessaries that can be placed into the vagina to support the bladder and other pelvic structures. (Figure 15.1 shows a number of different types.) No individual pessary has a particular advantage over others in general, but for a specific woman, one pessary may be preferable to another. The decision as to which one to use should be made by the physician at the time of the examination. For some women with moderate-sized cystoceles, a large tampon may suffice to offer support. These should be changed frequently because of the risk of infection associated with leaving a tampon in place for twelve to twenty-four hours. In general, pessaries should be removed once a week, cleaned, and replaced. Most women can be taught to do this themselves. If the woman is not on estrogen replacement therapy, the use of vaginal estrogen cream twice a week should be encouraged in order to keep the epithelium of the vagina as healthy as possible. Most women prefer to take baths or plain water douches to keep the area clean, and this can be done

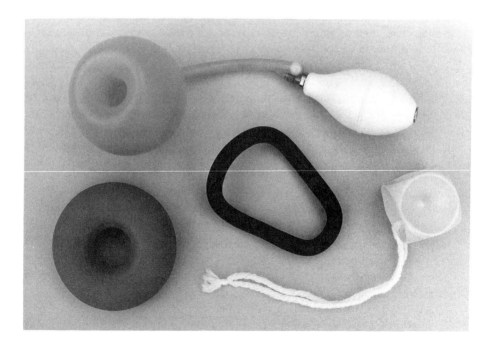

FIGURE 15.1.   A variety of pelvic pessaries.

every few days. Often pessaries will be expelled at the time of bowel movements or with straining. This can partially be avoided by holding the pessary in place while straining with stool. If the pessary is expelled, it can be washed and replaced without any harm being done. At times, after long use of pessaries, some erosion of the vaginal wall takes place, and bleeding may occur. This is not dangerous and does not indicate the development of a cancer. It is best treated by leaving the pessary out for a few days and treating the patient with vaginal estrogen cream to aid healing. Of course, a physician should examine the patient to be sure that this is the cause of the bleeding.

The surgical repair of a cystocele and urethrocele is generally done vaginally. In most cases, the defect is damage to the endopelvic fascia, and this can be repaired with an operation called an anterior colporrhaphy. In this operation, the vaginal epithelium is separated from the fascia, and sutures are placed in such a way as to pick up healthy areas laterally in the fascia and bring them to the midline. The procedure can be carried out over the urethra and urethrocele, if present, but in such instances attention must be paid to resupporting the bladder neck behind the pubic bone. This can be accomplished with a number of different procedures, but the actual approach in an individual patient should be left to the discretion of the surgeon who is aware of her specific needs. In the occasional case in which the endopelvic fascia is torn from the pelvic support structure laterally, a paravaginal repair can be performed. This is an abdominal procedure rather than a vaginal one and requires the suturing of the lateral endopelvic fascia supports to lateral pelvic structures.

After surgical repair of a cystocele, a Foley catheter is generally left in place for a few days, but it is then removed and the patient is evaluated for her ability to void and for a residual of urine that may be present in the bladder. If she can void and the residual urine is small, then no further catheter therapy is necessary. For a relatively small number of women, the reinstitution of voiding may be prolonged, and they may need to have catheter drainage for a few additional days. Given the fact that hospital stays are now short, it is possible for the woman to go home with the Foley catheter in place, attached to a leg bag, and return to her physician's office in a few days for removal.

Some physicians use a suprapubic catheter placed at the time of operation into the bladder and brought out through a stab incision in the abdominal wall. This allows for continuous drainage of the bladder, and after a few days the catheter can be clamped and the woman can attempt to void. Because the catheter is in the bladder, residual urines can be measured at that time. This does create added trauma to the bladder, and most surgeons will simply use drainage of the bladder in the traditional fashion.

Postoperative care is extremely important. Most surgeons use an absorbable suture that keeps its tensile strength for about one month. At the end of the month a great deal of healing has taken place, but the healing is not really completed for about three months or longer. Therefore, the woman should avoid straining, lifting, standing for long periods of time, and intercourse for at least three months in order to give the area a chance to heal. In my experience, most recurrent cystoceles take place not because the procedure was not done correctly but because the woman did not allow enough time for healing before resuming normal activities. This was more common in the days when absorbable suture had sufficient tensile strength of only about a week. Fortunately, newer sutures are available that have helped to alleviate this problem.

CASE STUDY

June is a fifty-year-old married woman with four children and is currently peri-menopausal. Her periods have been irregular, but they are still occurring. She had a large cystocele and rectocele as well as a uterine prolapse, and she underwent a vaginal hysterectomy and anterior and posterior colporrhaphy eighteen months ago by another physician. She and her husband like to ride motorcycles and belong to a motorcycle club of people in their age group who often take weekend trips together. They are sexually active and have intercourse on an average of four to five times a week.

When I examined June, I found that she had a large recurrent cystocele but did not seem to have a rectocele or any other evidence for prolapse. I reviewed the operative note of her first surgeon and found that her repair was done with suture material that was absorbable and had a tensile strength sufficient for about seven days. Furthermore, June said that she was told that after six weeks she could resume her normal activities. In her case, this consisted of riding a motorcycle and having frequent intercourse. She noticed a recurrence of her cystocele shortly thereafter; it had gotten larger and now protruded through the introitus. She did not have any incontinence.

I performed a simple cystocele repair (anterior colporrhaphy) using a suture, although absorbable, that continued its tensile strength for about a month. I also instructed June not to have intercourse and not to ride a motorcycle for three months.

With these precautions, she healed well and has enjoyed good health, and has had no recurrence of her cystocele.

RECTOCELE

Like a cystocele, the rectocele is a bulge into the vagina, except that it is on the posterior wall. The woman may complain of heaviness in the pelvis or a sensation that her rectum is falling out of her vagina. She may have constipation and occasionally state that she needs to splint her vagina with her fingers in order to effect a bowel movement. She may have the feeling of incomplete emptying of the rectum after a bowel movement.

The rectocele can be seen on vaginal examination with the woman in stirrups, but it should be examined with her standing as well as lying down. At the time of the examination, the physician will attempt to decide whether or not the bulge is simply a rectocele or rectocele and enterocele. This is important to know as the surgeon plans therapy for the patient. The examination is generally carried out with the surgeon having one finger in the rectum and one finger in the vagina. In this way, the rectocele can be identified and the surgeon can note the sensation of a bulge above the rectocele that may signal an enterocele.

Like the cystocele, the rectocele may first be treated with nonsurgical methods, including estrogen and possibly a pessary. If the woman has a good perineal body, that is, the area between the rectum and the posterior vaginal opening, where a number of the superficial diaphragm muscles come together, the pessary should be held in place without difficulty. In this way the woman may be kept comfortable so that estrogen and Kegel exercise use may give the physician some idea of the amount of resolution that will take place without surgery. On the other hand, some women with pelvic relaxation problems, including rectocele, will have a poor perineal body, usually secondary to the trauma of giving birth. In this case, they may have difficulty holding a pessary in place, and the need for surgery may be apparent earlier.

The surgical repair procedure consists of a posterior colporrhaphy. In this case, the vaginal epithelium is separated from the rectum and the levator ani muscles are identified, mobilized laterally, and brought together in the midline between the rectum and the vagina. I like to use permanent suture, that is, one that will not be resorbed, in order to give this area strength and stability over a long period of time. At the time of the rectocele repair, it is again important to look for evidence of an enterocele. With the vaginal epithelium separated, it is possible to see the hernia sac of an enterocele protruding from the abdominal cavity. If this is found, it can be repaired at the same time. Following a rectocele repair, it is equally important that the woman refrain from lifting, stretching, or intercourse for about three months. The stool should be kept soft with a stool softener so that constipation and straining do not occur. If the perineal body is inadequate, it can be repaired at the time of the posterior colporrhaphy. This procedure, perineorrhaphy, consists primarily of bringing the muscle bundles of the superficial compartment together in the midline, thereby building up the perineum once again.

It is unusual to repair only a rectocele or a cystocele unless previous repairs have taken place. In general, if there is a need for a cystocele repair, there is also a need for a rectocele repair and vice versa. Strengthening one wall of the vagina will often cause relaxation of the other wall even though it may have appeared reasonably healthy to start with. Therefore, in patients with pelvic relaxation, we almost always perform a cystocele and rectocele repair at the same time. Not to do so often means that the woman will need another operation in six months to one year.

CASE STUDY

Penny is sixty-three years old. When she was fifty, she underwent a vaginal hysterectomy and anterior colporrhaphy because of bleeding and stress incontinence. At the time her physician did not see an obvious rectocele, and no repair was done. For about the past ten to twelve years she has had an increasing bulge in the posterior wall of her vagina. At times, it bulges through the introitus. For several months she has had to splint her vaginal wall in order to have a bowel movement. She has been severely constipated and has had to use cathartics and enemas to obtain relief. Penny is five feet, three inches tall and weighs 200 pounds. She has been a smoker all of her life and smokes about a pack of cigarettes per day. She has a chronic cough.

(continued)

CASE STUDY (CONTINUED)

Upon examination, I noted a huge rectocele that with straining bulged through the introitus. When a finger was placed in her rectum, the rectal and vaginal walls were noted to be extremely thin. A rectocele repair was performed. Postoperatively she was placed on a high-fiber diet, encouraged to drink large amounts of fluid, and was given a mild bulk laxative. She has done well for the two years since her surgery without any evidence of recurrence of her rectocele.

Penny is a good example of someone with a weakened posterior vaginal wall that became worse over the years. Her obesity and poor diet habits contributed to her constipation, which probably made her problem worse. Therapy consisted of not only an anatomical repair but also of improving her diet by adding more fiber and more liquid to decrease the chance of constipation. A mild cathartic was also felt to be necessary.

ENTEROCELE

An enterocele is a true hernia of the peritoneal cavity into the posterior vaginal region. In the posterior area of the pelvis behind the cervix and between the uterosacral ligaments, there is only vaginal epithelium and peritoneum between the peritoneal cavity and the vagina. If this area stretches, as with weakening of the uterosacral ligaments, it forms a potential space through which a hernia can begin to descend. Since the hernia sac that will develop is covered with the peritoneal lining of the abdominal cavity and the vagina, it is a true hernia. It often contains small bowel. Occasionally it can contain other structures, such as a prolapsed ovary, omentum, or even a loop of sigmoid colon. The symptoms will be a bulge in the posterior vaginal wall, and it may be difficult to differentiate this from a rectocele. Often, both are present. However, as the enterocele enlarges, it will push through the vaginal opening and protrude. When the sac is palpated, small bowel loops will be felt. Some surgeons will transilluminate the sac with a flashlight and actually see the loops of bowel within it. Often, in older patients with total prolapse and large enteroceles, the vaginal epithelium will be ulcerated. It is difficult to repair such a hernia until the epithelium is healthy. Therefore, pessaries may help to hold the sac inside the vagina, and estrogen creams may help the healing process. It may take a few months for this to heal before an operation may be performed. Enteroceles can occur with the uterus in place; but often they occur following a hysterectomy. Since an enterocele is a hernia, the bowel within the sac may become strangulated, and the woman may first be seen as having an acute abdominal emergency.

Enteroceles that have not been previously repaired can be repaired vaginally. With the vaginal epithelium opened, it is possible to identify the sac, dissect it free of the vaginal wall and rectum, isolate the neck of the sac as it comes from the abdominal cavity, empty the sac of its contents (bowel, and so on), and then plicate the neck of the sac with sutures, following which the sac wall is trimmed away. It is important to reinforce the area through which the sac protruded, and this is often done as part of the rectocele repair that usually accompanies an enterocele repair, bringing the levator ani muscles together as high as possible. In women who have no rectocele, usually due to previous surgery, but do have an enterocele, it is possible to continue the old rectocele repair higher in order to reinforce the area of the enterocele.

Repeat enteroceles or very large enteroceles can be repaired abdominally. I often use an abdominal and vaginal approach. After the sac is dissected free, its neck sutured, and the tissue trimmed away, I usually obliterate the lower area of the abdominal cavity, known as the cul-de-sac, with consecutive layers of silk sutures. This essentially elevates the pelvic floor and removes the pressure of bowel into the weakened area next to the vagina. The enterocele may also be repaired from above only by elevating the sac into the abdominal cavity, plicating its neck, and then performing an obliteration of the cul-de-sac. The choice of operation should be left to the surgeon, since each case is quite different and should individualized. I am often referred patients who have a preconceived notion of what I will do. I find each case to be different and the repair to actually pose an engineering problem. I generally think about the anatomy and the type of defect for a few weeks before deciding upon the type of procedure I will employ. If you suffer from such a problem, I believe it is important to work with your physician to arrive at a solution that is specifically appropriate for you. Occasionally, if the defect is large enough, it is necessary to reinforce the pelvic floor with an inert material such as mersilene. This is often necessary for women who have been operated upon many times and who are usually obese or suffer from chronic cough. This is a circumstance that should be looked at individually and decided upon in consultation with your physician.

UTERINE PROLAPSE

Uterine prolapse is the protrusion of the cervix and uterus down the vaginal canal and possibly through the vaginal opening. A first-degree prolapse is a movement of the cervix and uterus down the upper third of the vagina. A second-degree prolapse is a prolapse that is lower into the vagina but not through the introitus. A third-degree prolapse, sometimes known as total (complete) prolapse, occurs when the cervix and uterus are completely through the vaginal opening. Prolapses are frequently associated with other pelvic relaxation problems such as cystocle and rectocele. While they may occur because of congenital weakening or absence of various pelvic support structures, they are most often seen in women who have had children. These women complain of a heaviness in the pelvis. If it is an advanced second-degree prolapse, a woman may note a bulge inside her introitus when she strains. If it is a total prolapse, she will note a mass protruding from the vagina. If this is left unchecked, ulcerations of the cervix and the vagina may occur, and there may be bleeding and pain.

As with other pelvic relaxation problems, it is prudent to treat such a woman with estrogen replacement therapy if they have not yet taken it and to use a pessary in the meantime to effect support. Certainly if there are ulcerations this must be done in conjunction with vaginal estrogen cream to effect healing before any surgical procedures can be considered. After a few months, when the maximum results of estrogen replacement therapy and pelvic exercises are realized, the woman may be considered for surgery.

A variety of procedures can be offered, depending upon the woman's health and age as much as anything else. For younger women, the standard treatment is a vaginal hysterectomy, usually in conjunction with an anterior and posterior colporrhaphy since a cystocele and rectocele are almost always present as well. Other operations can be used. One of these is a Manchester procedure, which involves the amputation of the cervix and the utilization of the cervical supporting ligaments, the cardinal ligaments, in the repair. Anterior and posterior colporrhaphies are performed in conjunction with this procedure. The operation was originally developed in England to save a younger woman's fertility if she had a uterine prolapse. However, it requires the partial or complete removal of the cervix, and this will often lead to an incompetent cervix and miscarriage in women who are still in their reproductive years. It does have an application in older women who wish to retain their uterus or who do not wish to undergo a more invasive procedure of a hysterectomy. Long-term satisfactory results are similar for this procedure and for vaginal hysterectomy. It is particularly of help for elderly women who often have a long cervix that appears to be prolapsing without significant prolapse of the uterus itself. In such cases, it allows for a relatively short procedure with excellent results.

In very elderly women or women who are in extremely poor health and are not likely to be sexually active in the future, it is possible to perform a procedure that essentially closes the vagina. This procedure is known as a colpocleisis, and the commonest variation is one that was developed by a gynecologist named L. LeFort and bears his name. In this procedure a large strip of vaginal epithelium is removed from both the anterior and posterior vaginal walls, and then the walls are sutured together, essentially closing down the vagina. If the uterus is still present, the small passageway on each side of the vagina is left open. Should the woman have uterine bleeding, it would be detectable. The cervix, however, is covered by the vaginal closure, and the use of Pap smears is usually impossible except for scrapings of the lateral vaginal walls. The operation is generally performed in conjunction with a plication of the bladder neck to try to prevent urinary incontinence, and if an enterocele is found to be present, it must be repaired. This procedure will often give satisfactory results with respect to a prolapse. It may be used in situations in which the uterus is already removed to close down the remaining vagina, and it can be performed under local anesthesia if the woman is in very poor health.

PROLAPSE OF THE VAGINAL STUMP

For the woman who has had a previous hysterectomy and now has a prolapse of the vaginal stump, a number of procedures to suspend the vagina are possible. The vagina may be suspended to a pelvic ligament known as the sacrospinus ligament. This is a vaginal procedure. The vagina may also be suspended to a part of the lower back known as the sacrum, but this is an abdominal procedure and often requires the use of an inert stent generally made of mersilene, since it is not likely that in most women that the vaginal wall will be long enough to reach to the sacrum. Many prolapses of the vagina after a hysterectomy are due to an enterocele. Repairing the enterocele alone is usually all that is required, although physicians may desire to suspend the vagina as well as a safety precaution.

Prolapses of the vaginal vault after previous hysterectomy should be carefully evaluated and the appropriate operation designed by the surgeon after taking into consideration all of the anatomical factors. As with all other pelvic relaxation problems, the use of estrogen and a pessary can be applied prior to surgery or instead of surgery in some individual cases. If the prolapsed vagina is ulcerated, this therapy must be undertaken in order to heal the ulcers before surgery is attempted.

CASE STUDY

Mary is an eighty-year-old widow who has mild coronary artery disease and high blood pressure, both of which are adequately treated at the present time. She underwent a hysterectomy for a fibroid uterus at age forty-nine and never took hormone replacement therapy. For the past two years, she has had a prolapse of her vagina but has supported it until recently with a Kotex pad. She did not consult a physician. Recently the prolapse has become more severe, and the Kotex pad does not hold it back. She has also noted some vaginal bleeding and therefore consulted her gynecologist. She was found to have a total prolapse of the vaginal vault and a cystocele, rectocele, and enterocele. There were ulcerations of the vaginal epithelium that appeared clean but bled on touch. Her gynecologist performed biopsies of the ulcers, which proved to be benign. She was given a pessary and prescribed estrogen cream, and after two months the ulcers were healed. Since she was widowed, not sexually active, and in moderate health, her physician suggested a colpocleisis of the LeFort type. Mary consented. Since she was not incontinent, her physician felt that he could fix the enterocele and perform the colpocleisis in relatively short operative time. The day before the surgery was scheduled, Mary called the physician and stated that she had a dream that her dead husband had returned and was concerned that she no longer had a vagina. Her gynecologist realized that Mary had had second thoughts about losing her vagina and asked her if she would rather have a repair of the defect without closing the vagina. She stated that she would.

The next day she underwent a cystocele, rectocele, and enterocele repair and a suspension of her vaginal vault. She went through the surgery without any complications and has had a good anatomical result postoperatively.

This case illustrates the fact that even though a woman may be widowed and no longer sexually active, may be older and in less than good health, she may have feelings that need to be taken into consideration in planning the procedure she will undergo. In this case, Mary's health was good enough for her to tolerate a more extensive procedure, and her physician was sensitive enough to understand her desires.

CASE STUDY

Greta is ninety-one years old and is in reasonably good health except for the fact that she has severe Alzheimer's disease and has been living in a nursing home for the past six years. She is incontinent and had a total prolapse of her vagina, which is ulcerated. She was referred to my office by her son, who is seventy years old. She did not recognize him, though strangely enough she remembered me from previous visits.

After examining her, I realized she had a prolapse of the vagina and an enterocele but also had relaxation of the bladder neck. Apparently her urinary incontinence was causing a nursing problem in the home where she resides. I told her son that it was not possible to determine whether or not surgical repair would relieve her incontinence, as part of it may have been due to her mental status. He discussed this at the nursing home with the nurses, who were anxious for me to do whatever I could to help alleviate the problem. Therefore, I performed an operation in which I supported the bladder neck, did an enterocele repair, and a colpocleisis of the LeFort type. The patient got a nice anatomical result, and the nurses at the nursing home reported that her incontinence was improved during the day but that she still wet the bed during the night. They were, however, grateful for the improvement.

This Alzheimer's patient had severe nursing problems, but she also had anatomical defects that could, at least in part, be alleviated surgically. It is difficult to assess how much of her dignity was restored, but her caregivers believed that she was happier after having had the procedure. Her decrease in incontinence during waking hours seemed to support this.

CONCLUSIONS

There are many types of problems related to relaxation or damage to pelvic support structures. For each individual case, the physician must perform a careful examination and evaluation to determine the anatomical defect and design an operation that fits the needs of the woman and her long-term requirements. Since these support structures are estrogen sensitive, estrogen replacement therapy should be used whenever possible. In many cases the patient would benefit from muscle exercises even if surgery were going to be performed, but I cannot stress enough the need to individualize therapy for each specific woman, based upon her individual needs.

CHAPTER 16

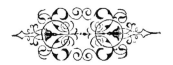

Grief and Loss: How to Deal with It and Survive

Everyone suffers losses throughout a lifetime. For young women it may be the ending of a relationship, the loss of a friend or a relative by separation or death, infertility problems, miscarriage, the loss of a job, or the loss of a pet. For older women, the losses tend to pile up and include not only the loss of friends and relatives through separation or death, or the loss of a spouse to divorce or death, but also may include loss of children, jobs, the ability to participate in sports or other activities, the loss of body organs, and of pets. The loss of pets is not a frivolous matter, as some elderly people may have very little other contact with living or loving beings.

Losses of all sorts can produce a grief reaction. This is usually accompanied by both physical and emotional symptoms. In the mid 1940s Lindemann, a psychiatrist, described the grief reaction as a tightness in the throat and chest, a choking sensation, shortness of breath, frequent sighing, an empty feeling in the abdomen, muscle weakness, a feeling of tension and mental pain, and guilt (see Table 16.1). Any or all of these symptoms usually occur acutely after a loss. The symptoms will frequently go on for as long as six months to two years, depending upon the ability of the woman to replace her loss with other individuals or activities. For the very elderly who may have very few opportunities to replace whatever has been lost, the grieving process may go on a great deal longer. In addition, there are many cultural variations in the grieving process that may influence how and for how long a person grieves.

One of the most severe losses that a woman suffers is the death of a child. It can create such a severe grief reaction that it may last for a prolonged period of time, but it may be modified by the presence of other children in the home or by new pregnancies. Older women, however, are often faced with the death of an adult child. In wartime, this occurs when young men become battle casualties or when children are lost during bombing attacks or other acts of war. Recently, however, a new killer of young people, the AIDS epidemic, has become common. Many young adults with HIV will be cared for by their mothers throughout their prolonged illness and until

TABLE 16.1.   Grief Reaction

Tightness in throat and chest

Choking sensation

Shortness of breath

Frequent sighing

Empty feeling in the abdomen

Muscle weakness

Feeling of tension and mental pain

Guilt

TABLE 16.2.   Morbid Grief

Delay of reaction

Distorted reaction

Psychosomatic conditions

Pathologic alterations of relationships

Inappropriate behavior pattern

Psychotic behavior pattern

Inability to make decisions or take initiative

Social or economic destructiveness

Agitated depression (suicide)

their death. Therefore, the mothers will suffer the loss of a child and will also need to deal with a prolonged process of dying associated with this condition. Generally, the grief reaction in these women is very acute, and its length and depth will depend a great deal on other factors in the woman's life.

The loss of a spouse through death or divorce will usually increase psychological distress. The type of emotional problems that a woman will have generally follow her usual behavior pattern. If she has been an anxious person or has suffered from depression, the symptoms will usually become more acute.

MORBID GRIEF

Lindemann also described a number of situations in which grief reaction was abnormal and could, in many cases, have serious consequences for the individual. (See Table 16.2.)

The delay of reaction is a very interesting phenomena. Generally, it is seen when the patient herself is in a life-threatening situation and does not seem to grieve appropriately for the loss of a loved one. For instance, if a couple is in a motor vehicle accident and the husband is killed and the wife seriously injured, the wife may not seem to grieve when she is told that her husband is dead. She may demonstrate a full-blown grief reaction six months later when she is healed. To the casual observer, this response to a loss that occurred six months earlier seems inappropriate, but it can be looked upon as occurring only when she has the emotional energy to enter into the grief reaction.

CASE STUDY

Irene is a patient of mine who demonstrated a delay of grief reaction. She was fifty-five years old and had just been diagnosed as having ovarian cancer. Fortunately, her disease was picked up early, and we performed appropriate surgery. On her second postoperative day, Irene's husband died of an acute heart attack on his way to work. My social worker and I broke the news to her, and she seemed to take it very well. She made comments like "Yes, he had a bad heart" and "I am glad he did not suffer." On the other hand, she did not cry or show any other signs of an acute grief reaction. We suspected that she might be in a delay of reaction and were not surprised when three weeks later, after she had been discharged from the hospital and was in the process of making an uneventful recovery, her son called to state that she was sobbing inconsolably and manifesting several symptoms of an acute grief reaction.

Clearly, Irene looked upon her cancer as an extremely serious event in her life, and she was not able to grieve for her husband until she realized that she would probably survive.

The distorted reaction is seen frequently in an adult daughter who has lost a mother to whom she was close. She may not show evidence of a grief reaction but takes on mannerisms of the deceased. She may comb her hair, wear clothes, and walk like the deceased person. If the person who died had symptoms of an illness prior to death, the survivor may even take on the symptoms of the deceased. This reaction may go on for some time, but generally she will eventually grieve and then return to her own normal behavior pattern. During the time of the distorted reaction, the woman often believes that she sees an image of the deceased or that she sees people in crowds that resemble the deceased. This symptom is not necessarily specific to the distorted reaction, as it is often noted by the newly bereaved as well.

People who have illnesses that are thought to have a psychosomatic component, such as asthma, ulcerative colitis, or rheumatoid arthritis, will often have a flare-up of symptoms at the time of a loss. It is important for their family members and physicians to expect a flare-up of the condition under the stress of grief.

Pathologic alterations of relationships are frequently seen in the bereaved. Relationships with friends or relatives may be altered, the bereaved may blame others for the death, or a relationship may be altered because of the guilt felt by the bereaved. Children in the family are often the targets of this behavior. The extreme may be the blame placed by a father on a child whose mother died giving birth.

Inappropriate behavior patterns are frequently seen in those suffering from an abnormal grief reaction, who may develop inappropriate fears such as being afraid to leave the house, believing others are trying to harm them, or fearing driving a car. They may develop compulsions requiring them to act out certain behavior patterns, such as tapping the wall a certain number of times as they walk from room to room. They may have difficulty sleeping and may walk the streets at night without any obvious purpose. A huge variety of abnormal behaviors have been seen in such people.

An extreme is the development of psychotic behavior patterns. In such a situation, a person may hear voices telling her to act out certain imagined commands, or she may sit for long periods of time staring blankly at a wall. Those with a previous tendency toward psychotic behavior are more susceptible, but this problem has been seen in otherwise previously normal-appearing individuals.

The inability to make decisions or take initiatives is quite frequent and may last for a year or two after the loss of a loved one. This is often seen in widows who are suddenly expected to manage family assets. They often become susceptible to predators, including people who have been close to them.

CASE STUDY

Marilyn is a sixty-one-year-old physician's wife. Her husband recently died of cancer, leaving her with a large farm, a cabin near a ski resort, and a twenty-one-foot power boat. Marilyn and her husband had enjoyed these things together. Their three children were grown and had left the area. One evening, shortly after her husband's death, a sister and her husband visited Marilyn and asked what she was planning to do with the power boat. She stated that she had not thought about it, and they immediately suggested that she probably would not need it anymore and offered her $800 to take it off her hands. The boat was relatively new and probably worth about $15,000. Marilyn consented, feeling that she would probably not use the boat any longer. Her sister and husband left that evening with the boat and its trailer.

When she visited my office a few weeks later, we discussed what had happened. I suggested that she might be preyed upon again, perhaps by people who had been close to her, and I warned her to be aware that this might happen. A few weeks later, a cousin and her husband approached her to buy her ski cabin. Again, a ridiculously low price was offered after several sympathetic words about her lost husband and her bereavement. Marilyn politely declined the offer and was surprised to see how quickly the couple's attitude toward her changed.

(continued)

CASE STUDY (CONTINUED)

They asked what she could possibly do with such a cabin now that she was a widow, and abruptly left. Marilyn then consulted her accountant, got a breakdown of what her net worth was and of the properties she owned, and decided not to make any financial decisions with respect to her property for at least one year.

This was a wise decision. I recommend to all of my patients who are recently widowed not to make any financial decisions they may regret. Before making any financial decisions, if you are recently widowed, get an accounting of your worth, and put off deciding how you will deal with it until you are functioning appropriately.

SOCIAL OR ECONOMIC DESTRUCTIVENESS

Although this abnormal grief reaction is similar to some of the other items mentioned, it usually involves a more active destructiveness. The grieving woman may sign all of her property over to children or family members, get in her car, and drive away to a distant city, essentially abandoning everything she and her husband worked for. This type of reaction is often seen with divorce, but it can also occur with death.

CASE STUDY

Imogene and her husband owned a small farm on which they worked together. They had no children, and she was fifty-five years old. One day she returned home earlier than expected from a trip to the local city and found her husband in bed with her sister. She packed a small suitcase, got in her car, and drove two thousand miles across the country from Washington State to Pennsylvania. She had no friends or relatives in Pennsylvania, but she came across a small town near Harrisburg that she rather fancied. She got a job as a waitress in a small restaurant and began her life all over. She never contacted anyone, and her husband, in whose name the farm was owned, sold the farm and took all of their assets.

While the grief reaction she suffered after discovering her husband's lack of faithfulness and the involvement of her sister was understandable, in the long run she lost her place in the society she had grown up in and all of her economic security.

Agitated depression is probably the most dangerous reaction. It is often seen when a mother loses a child, but it occurs as a reaction to other losses as well. The person becomes despondent and agitated. She cannot sleep, guilt and anger become mixed in her thought process, and her depression is usually acute and deep. It is not uncommon that such a person commits suicide.

LOSS OF AN ORGAN OR OTHER BODY PART

Loss of a body part or vital organ can be expected to bring about a grief reaction, with accompanying symptoms of both an emotional and physical nature. Depression is frequently a strong component. It is often seen with the loss of limbs, an eye, or a body part that is part of the woman's identity, such as a breast, uterus, or ovaries. Several different studies have demonstrated depression in posthysterectomy patients, and the incidence has been reported to vary from 4 to 70 percent, depending upon how well prepared the woman was for the surgery.

Several years ago, an investigator named Roberts suggested that there were four stages of incorporation that a patient needed to go through to accept the loss of an important body part. These were: impact, retreat, acknowledgment, and reconstruction.

During the impact period, the woman may not even hear that an organ needs to be removed. She may actually deny that such information was given. She may not be able, at that time, to incorporate such a piece of information into her thought process. Generally, the physician will need to repeat the recommendation on more than one occasion.

The retreat aspect usually involves the person's desire to find an alternative to this recommendation. Therefore, second opinions are often sought from other physicians. This is healthy and should be encouraged so that the person is satisfied, when the time comes, that the right decision has been made. During this time she will seek alternatives of therapy. This too is healthy unless it is carried to an extreme. For instance, a cancer patient may prolong the period between diagnosis and treatment by seeking alternative therapies that she finds more acceptable. During that time, the disease may pass beyond a curable stage.

Acknowledgment occurs when the person accepts the fact that the organ will be removed but asks many questions about how the procedure will be performed, the type of anesthesia used, the length of the hospital stay, the way she will feel after the operation, and the time she will miss from work or other activities.

The reconstruction phase involves questions about what she will be like after the procedure has been performed, and how others will respond to her. In the case of a woman who is undergoing a hysterectomy, she may wish to know what she will be like sexually after the procedure and how she may expect her husband to relate to her. In such matters it is important to involve both members of the couple in these discussions so that no inappropriate fantasies are harbored.

If the woman goes through all of these stages before the procedure is performed, the risk of depression and grief after the procedure is lessened. If she is rushed into surgery either because of the emergent nature of her disease or because of scheduling considerations, she may not have time to work through these steps and may suffer a fairly acute and prolonged grief reaction.

LOSS OF A PET

Although on the surface this may sound frivolous, pets are very important in the lives of many people. In the case of many older women who lead a fairly isolated life with rare contacts with other people, the pet may be the only living creature in their day-to-day existence. Thus, the loss of that pet may provoke an acute grief reaction. If this occurs, the woman should be encouraged to get another pet when she is ready. Physicians, friends, and relatives should not be surprised at her reactions. Of course, not all pet loss problems are seen in older people.

CASE STUDY

Susan is a second-year resident in obstetrics and gynecology. She and her husband own a few acres of land and had two pet sheep that they had raised from lambs. Susan and I were attending a medical meeting in a distant city when her husband called to tell her that a drunken driver had driven up on their property and struck both sheep, killing them instantly. Susan was devastated. She sobbed uncontrollably and then related many stories about her sheep when they were babies and how she had raised them. She demonstrated as acute a grief reaction from the loss as I have seen. Fortunately, after several weeks, a neighbor presented the couple with two baby lambs, and gradually Susan's grief abated.

LOSS OF A JOB

The loss of a job is devastating to anyone, as it implies failure. To an older person it is doubly difficult because the job may not be easily replaced. Also, she may have lost her job because of her age. Even though age discrimination is illegal in the United States, it can and does occur.

CASE STUDY

Geraldine was a sixty-year-old divorced woman who had been an accountant at a small manufacturing firm for the past fifteen years. Recently her boss had been promoted and replaced in her office by a younger man who made increasingly greater demands on her, and she found herself working ten to twelve hours per day to keep up with them. She began to suffer from anxiety and depression, and the manifestations of this affected her work, causing her employer to place even greater pressure upon her. After about eighteen months, she was told that her job was being discontinued, and she was laid off. She had saved a small amount of money, but she was angry because she had not planned to stop working, and because stopping at this point two years short of her being eligible for Social Security placed her in some financial difficulty.

(continued)

CASE STUDY (CONTINUED)

When she consulted me she was complaining of tightness in her chest, palpitations, occasional bouts of shortness of breath, and a feeling of weakness. She was having difficulty sleeping and asked me for sleeping pills. She was also worried that she was developing a heart condition. While discussing her problems with me, she sighed a great deal and became tearful whenever she mentioned her job.

Her physical examination and appropriate laboratory studies were all normal. It was clear to me that she was suffering a grief reaction, and we discussed this at length. Fortunately she had a great deal of spirit, and when she realized that she was not ill, she was able to find some part-time work that got her out of the house and improved her finances.

Some women are fortunate enough to find other work or outside activities. The degree of the grief reaction will probably be more severe in women who do not have a large number of options.

IMPENDING DEATH

In 1969 Elizabeth Kubler-Ross revolutionized our thinking about death by pointing out that death has always been distasteful and, in the minds of most people, is never considered possible in regard to themselves. She pointed out that in the simplest terms in our unconscious minds, we can only be killed. It is inconceivable for us to die of a natural cause or old age. Therefore, we look upon death as a bad act, a frightening happening, something that in itself calls for retribution and punishment.

Kubler-Ross described five stages through which a person progresses in acceptance of the inevitability of death. These are: denial, anger, bargaining, depression, and acceptance.

The denial stage is usually temporary and is brought about by the shock of learning that the person suffers from a problem from which she cannot recover. As with the information regarding the loss of an organ, frequently she will need to be told of this circumstance on several occasions. Transition to partial acceptance depends upon the nature of the illness and upon the amount of time she has left before death is expected to occur. It also probably depends upon the way in which she has been prepared through life to cope with a serious illness. In the early stages, it is natural for her to go through the denial phase by seeking multiple opinions from other physicians. This is a very healthy activity and should be encouraged.

After the person has accepted the fact that death will occur in the foreseeable future, anger generally is the next stage. In this situation it is frequently difficult to deal with her, for both health care workers and the family. A physician may enter her room and state in a friendly, jovial manner that she is looking quite well today. She may angrily respond, "What, are you crazy? I am dying. How can I look well?" The next day the physician may enter the room in a more somber fashion and softly ask how she is feeling. The patient may then again angrily respond, "What kind of a crepe hanger are you; can't you be more cheerful?" Clearly, members of the family can be treated in the same fashion. Such behavior often drives others away from the sick person, which is of course the opposite of the reaction she is hoping for. At this point she needs the presence and understanding of her family and caregivers.

The next stage is bargaining. In this stage, the person essentially tries to put her life in order. She may again find her religious roots and may make peace with family members with whom she has been quarreling. She will usually see that her financial affairs are in order and that her will is up-to-date. The bargaining aspect from her standpoint is that if she does everything just right, perhaps she will get a reprieve, undoubtedly from God. There is a reward in this phase, in that she will often derive mental satisfaction from putting things in order.

Depression may occur at any time, and it may be deep enough to necessitate treatment. This depends primarily upon her personality and the way in which she copes with other problems in her life.

The final step is that of acceptance. If the person lives long enough, she will frequently get to this stage. People have speculated about the possibility that this may simply be a wearing down because of the symptoms of the disease and that death will be a relief. Kubler-Ross found in her studies, however, that many people achieved acceptance who were not suffering severe symptoms.

Everyone on this planet will die sooner or later, and everyone reading this book will probably experience these steps in one way or another, unless death is sudden. As Kubler-Ross has pointed out, for most people death is a bad act and a frightening happening. It is helpful for us to know about the stages of this process, since as we age we will probably be called upon to share such an event with others who are going through it.

CHAPTER 17

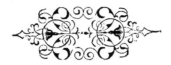

Depression, Dementia, Delirium:
What's the Difference?

Studies have shown that 50 to 60 percent of visits to primary care physicians are for complaints that have a behavioral or emotional component. Furthermore, about 25 percent of patients visiting primary care physicians or facilities have psychiatric disorders. Women suffer disproportionately from many of these conditions and have two to three times the risk for depression in their lifetime as do men.

Dementia, which involves the destruction of brain cells due to organic brain damage, is quite common in older people. Roughly 5 percent of people over the age of sixty-five have severe dementia, and 10 percent have mild dementia. After the age of eighty, a full 20 percent suffer from dementia.

Delirium is a disorder of brain physiology frequently due to other circumstances and is often reversible. Older women are very susceptible to depression, dementia, and the conditions leading to delirium; all of these will be discussed in this chapter.

THE AGING PROCESS

The aging process is associated with a slow diminution of physical ability. This has to do with a number of changes, including a decreased demineralization of bone, a decrease in muscle mass, a slow loss of heart and lung reserve, and the loss of the ability to detoxify substances due to a decrease in certain enzyme activity. Coupled with this, women also suffer the slow loss of sensory acuity affecting hearing, vision, sense of smell, and sense of taste. In addition, there is a weakening of connective tissue throughout the body due both to the lack of estrogen and to the other normal aging changes that take place.

Along with the physical changes, women must cope with a shift in their biological function from the reproductive mode to menopause. Since one third of a woman's life is generally spent after menopause, this shift can cause many repercussions.

Several brain function changes take place with the aging process. In general, knowledge acquired with socialization tends to remain stable, but the acquisition and retrieval of new information generally decreases. Along with this, creativity may decrease, although many older women are very creative. Problem-solving abilities decrease with age, giving the older person an appearance of having difficulty in making decisions, especially on a short-term basis. Along with this, there may be a decrease of fluidity of thought, the ability to move from one thought to another in a logical fashion without deviating to other ideas. Physiologically, what probably happens is that nerve impulses jump from one neuron to another, bringing in thoughts that are generally related but not necessarily directly so. As an example, I once asked a seventy-two-year-old woman how long she had been suffering with the abdominal pain that was the reason for her visit. She answered in the following fashion: "Well, doctor, I remember having the pain when I went to help my daughter in Denver, Colorado, after she gave birth to her third child. It was a very cold winter and we could not get out of the house for several days because of the snow and for two days the phone lines were down so we could not call anyone. Oh, yes, that was the year my granddaughter had the measles. . . . What was the question again, doctor?" This mental change is quite common in the elderly and may lead to people's becoming impatient with them. Physicians have learned to be patient and to gently redirect their thought process in order to gather needed information. Other people may not be quite as patient and may avoid these people because of their tendency to be talkative without direction.

Some of these changes that take place with the aging process may lead to self-image adjustment problems. Some women can handle these changes gracefully; others develop a great deal of stress because of them.

The aging process is also complicated by the interjection of the many occasions for grief. After sixty-five, widows outnumber widowers 5:1, a function of the fact that women tend to live longer than men. Grief situations are often brought about because of loss of other activities and abilities and because the loss involved may create social and financial problems that can add to the woman's emotional distress. The combination of these factors may be responsible for many physical and emotional symptoms.

DEPRESSION

Depression is quite common. It may be associated with bereavement, disappointment, or other types of loss. It is usually transient and frequently requires no therapy, although some of the milder antidepressant agents may be helpful in such situations when used for the short term. Generally kindness, social support, and understanding on the part of friends and family members as well as medical professionals is usually all that is necessary to get a woman through such circumstances. The problem may be more severe for those who are socially isolated. The cure for bereavement and loss is to replace what is lost with other social activities. Therefore, women suffering such losses should attempt to reach out to others rather than withdraw within themselves.

CASE STUDY

Teresa was fifty-six years old when her husband died following cardiac bypass surgery. Her only son lived in a different region of the country, two thousand miles away, and was unmarried. Teresa had always been a homemaker and had very few skills that would allow her to be employable. She lived in a small two-bedroom house, and she and her husband had always stayed to themselves, having very little interaction with their neighbors. She did not belong to any clubs or social groups, and she did not belong to a church. The couple had some savings, and her husband had enough insurance so that she could live modestly without very many frills.

Two months after her husband died, Teresa consulted her primary care physician because of chest pain, bouts of shortness of breath, and muscle weakness. She stated that she had not been eating well and that she had been having difficulty sleeping. She appeared tired and somewhat depressed. Her physician's physical and laboratory evaluation could not detect any serious pathology, and he diagnosed her condition as mild depression following bereavement. He prescribed a mild antidepressant medication but also asked her to meet in his clinic, with the social worker who readily ascertained that Teresa did not have a serious financial problem, although certainly she was not well off. She ascertained that she liked to cook and that she had an interest in young children. She was encouraged to pursue these areas and was able to find two part-time jobs, one with a catering agency, and the second with a day care center. Neither job paid a great deal, but they did help to supplement her income. Through these two activities, she met other women with similar needs and thus found a few friends that she could socialize with. Within six months she was feeling much better and no longer had a need for antidepressant medications. Life now had a purpose.

Teresa's case is an example of a mild depression disorder secondary to bereavement. Although she required medication to slow her slip into a deeper depression, with direction she was able to find other activities in her life to replace her loss.

Minor depression is very common particularly after bereavement or loss. It often is the result of a major change in direction of a woman's life necessitated by the loss. The thing to remember is that the only way to overcome loss is to find replacements in your life to fill the void left by what is lost. Replacement activities can be found in a number of places: a job, volunteer work, church work, pursuing hobbies, returning to school either for retraining or to increase your knowledge base, travel, or pursuing family activities. All of these are healthy directions to pursue, but those that are best for each person depend upon her individual needs and opportunities. They all represent a turning outward rather than a turning into oneself. Medication should not be relied upon for the long term in such situations, but should be utilized only as a bridge to get to other activities. Bereavement often is associated with thought and behavior disruptions, and it may be difficult to establish new goals and activities at a time closely related to the loss. Sympathetic friends and relatives or health care workers can be helpful in pointing out new directions, and their services should be utilized when necessary. The major point is to find directions which will help the woman turn outward rather than into herself. Turning inward can lead to a deepening of the depression.

Major depression is a different story. Roughly 5 percent of people attending primary care clinics have major depression disorders. This is about as common as high blood pressure. Women have about a 20 percent chance of having a major depression disorder at some time during their life. Depressed women are easy to identify. They appear tired, sad, and disinterested. They often speak slowly, have difficulty concentrating, and answer questions after several seconds of delay. Not everyone fits this picture, however. Many can put on a good front when they need to or can disguise their depression with other symptoms or complaints. Studies have shown that the diagnosis of depression is missed in primary care clinics as often as 50 to 90 percent of the time.

There are several screening techniques for diagnosing depression. The American Psychiatric Association has developed a diagnostic manual for mental disorders that offers criteria for diagnosing major depression. (See Table 17.1.) The presence of five or more of the items mentioned is considered indicative of major depressive disorder. The first two, depressed mood and loss of interest or pleasure in most activities, are considered the most serious symptoms of depression.

Many people with severe depression complain of physical symptoms that are medically unexplained, including headache, abdominal pain, chronic fatigue, backache, and gastrointestinal difficulties. Research has shown that about 50 percent of those who are finally found to have a major depressive disorder come to their physicians with physical complaints. This is a particularly common finding in women who

TABLE 17.1.   Major Depressive Disorder: Diagnosis Criteria

1. Depressed mood

2. Loss of interest or pleasure in most activities

3. Significant weight loss or gain; change in appetite

4. Insomnia or the need for excessive sleep

5. Muscle weakness or agitation

6. Fatigue or energy loss

7. Feelings of worthlessness

8. Guilt

9. Diminished ability to think or concentrate

10. Recurrent thoughts of death or suicide

are approaching menopause. Although menopausal women are no more likely to have a major depressive disorder than are premenopausal women, the adjustment to menopause is frequently difficult enough to bring to the surface the symptoms of major depression in a woman already suffering from this. I see many patients in my office who are referred because of difficulty with hormone regulation at the time of menopause. The general complaint is that after starting estrogen the patient felt well for a few weeks and then began to feel depressed. The amount of estrogen was frequently increased, which led to her feeling well again for a few more weeks, and then the depression returned. Many of these women feel that their problem is that they metabolize estrogen too rapidly. In truth, they metabolize estrogen just like everyone else; but estrogen is a mood elevator, and as with all other mood elevators, if it is being used for this purpose, larger and larger doses are necessary. On the other hand, large doses of estrogen are not physiologically safe, as they may cause hyperplasia of the endometrial lining of the uterus, reverse the cholesterol profile to favor LDL, and perhaps have a negative effect on the breasts. Therefore, it is important to keep the dose of estrogen at a proper physiological level and to determine whether or not a patient has a depression problem that itself may require treatment.

An important factor in the diagnosis of major depression is the necessity to define whether or not someone is suicidal. Physicians will often ask direct questions: "Have you thought about injuring yourself?" or "Have you thought about ending your life?" If a woman tells a physician that she has had such thoughts, the physician will generally ask how serious these thoughts have been and whether she has made any plans to put them into effect. During my interview with a fifty-two-year-old patient on her first visit, I became aware of the fact that she was suffering from a major depressive disorder. Her complaints were the need for hormone replacement therapy because of menopause, weight gain because of an increased appetite, difficulty sleeping, and the report of some hostility with her husband, who had a drinking problem. She actually appeared more angry than depressed. When I asked her about suicidal thoughts, she reached into her purse and produced a .38 caliber revolver, which she laid on the desk. She stated that she had thought about suicide and had purchased the gun for that purpose. She consented to an immediate psychiatric evaluation by a colleague and subsequently did well with antidepressant medications and a short course of psychotherapy. For my part, I once more saw the value of asking the proper questions.

There are three basic treatment models that may be used singly or in combination, depending upon individual needs. These are the medication, psychological, and social models. The medication model uses antidepressant drugs, powerful regulators of the nervous system that work directly on the junction of the neurons in the brain. Although all are effective, most have side effects, so the choice of the appropriate medication for an older woman must take these potential side effects into account. There are basically two general categories of medications; tricyclic drugs and the selective serotonin uptake inhibitors (SSRIs). Each works at the junction of the neurons but in a somewhat different fashion. Tricyclic medications include amitriptyline (Elavil), doxepin (Sinequain or Adepin), and imipramine (Tofranil). These medications usually have an anticholonergic effect, that is, they interfere with acetyl choline, the neurotransmitter of the parasympathetic nervous system. In older patients, they may cause dryness of the mouth, hesitancy in voiding, and, at times, delirium. Trazadone (Desyrel) is another such agent that has been known to cause a decrease in blood pressure. Occasionally patients will faint when they arise at night to void and may then suffer fractures because of falls induced by the fainting. However, many women can tolerate low doses of these agents, and the choice of whether or not to use them should be made in conjunction with their physician.

The newer SSRI drugs seem to be of value in treating depressive disorders in older patients. The common agents in this category are fluoxetine (Prozac), sertraline (Zoloft), and paroxetine (Paxil). These are fairly free of side effects, but they may depress the appetite somewhat, as may other antidepressant drugs. They may also have a mild effect on the desire component of sexuality. They can be used in much smaller doses than would be recommended for younger adults. For instance, the starting dose of Prozac for young people is 20 mg and of Zoloft is 50 mg. Older people can be started on 10 mg of Prozac and 25 mg of Zoloft. Some women will even do well on smaller doses. Doses can be increased over time until the desired effect is obtained. In general, it takes six weeks to reach a maintenance dose, and symptoms are generally not relieved for three to four weeks. A person who states that she feels much better after a week or two of therapy is probably getting a placebo effect. A true effect on depression takes a bit longer. Once she is started on an antidepressant, the woman should be followed by her physician at reasonable intervals (one to three months). If she is doing well, after six months to a year, it may be possible to taper off or stop the medication. People with a tendency to develop organic depression will often relapse and may need to be treated at successive intervals in the future.

The psychological treatment model consists of either psychotherapy or self-help therapy. It is aimed at problems the patient may be having that are related to the depression. These problems could be interpersonal relationships, problems with trust and coping, or difficulty in solving problems. Additional types of problems that would require psychotherapy or self-help therapy are a parental history of psychological disorders, history of alcohol abuse, personality disorders, or a history of emotional, physical, or sexual abuse. These conditions can have potent effects on emotional stability and may pose problems for many years. Therefore working them out with the aid of a therapist is a reasonable way of alleviating discomfort.

The social model utilizes the use of social services agencies or social workers. These are best consulted and their services utilized in situations in which domestic violence, severe financial difficulties, social isolation, bereavement, or decreasing functional ability seem to be problems. Ongoing domestic violence problems often require the services of a social service agency to direct women into safe situations and to aid with job training needs or financial difficulties when they occur because a woman leaves the abusive relationship. Women who are having financial difficulties can also be helped by social service agencies, perhaps to find them a place to stay, a means of making a living, or welfare assistance. Women who are socially isolated may be aided by social service agencies in finding groups that they can relate to. It may be possible to get them access to a food bank or, if they are disabled, access to a meals-on-wheels agency.

Social service workers can be very helpful in getting a patient through extensive bereavement. They can be equally helpful for disabled people, to find the resources they need to lead a reasonable life.

While the first line of treatment for severe depression is often medication, it is important for women to have their psychological and social needs met at the same time. Health care workers should be on the lookout for ways to aid their patients in these areas, but it is helpful if people realize that they can get this help when they need it and to understand the circumstances under which they really require it.

Psychosocial distress, complaints of anxiety, and depression are common reasons for seeing a health care worker. Many people, however, have been brought up to feel that depression or other emotional problems are a defect in their personality, a failure on their part, and therefore they are reluctant to reveal emotional symptoms. Frequently, they will somatize their symptoms and seek help for physical complaints. Physicians are trained to be aware of this, but every so often they will miss implications of depression. It is important to realize that organic depression is a brain function disorder, not a failure of social adjustment. It is an illness like any other and can cause severe disruption of life, even leading to death via suicide. Therefore, presenting the symptoms of depression to a health care worker should not be looked upon as a failure but rather as the reporting of an illness.

DEMENTIA

Mental impairment is common in elderly women. About 5 percent of the women over the age of sixty-five will have severe dementia, and 10 percent will have dementia of a milder nature. By age eighty, 20 percent of the population will have severe dementia. Dementia is caused by organic changes in the brain, and there are several different causes. In dementia, there is impairment of both short- and long-term memory. In addition, abstract thinking, the ability to consider and solve problems in a logical fashion, is impaired, as is judgment. Sufferers will often have difficulty putting their thoughts into words and may even have difficulty in speaking at all. Because the condition is due to brain cell damage, there may be motor problems relating to gait or the ability to perform tasks with the hands efficiently. Along with all of this, there are often personality changes.

TABLE 17.2.   Dementia: Destruction of Neurons

Alzheimer's disease

Multiple vascular infarcts

Advanced HIV

Chronic alcoholism

Creutzfelt-Jakob disease

Dementia is the result of the destruction of brain cells. The common causes are listed in Table 17.2. They include Alzheimer's disease, which is a degenerative disease of neurons, multiple infarcts caused by vascular accidents and strokes in which nerve cells are damaged, advanced infection with the human immunodeficiency virus (HIV), destruction of brain cells seen with chronic alcoholism or other drug use, and a viral condition known as Creutzfeldt-Jakob disease in which the virus attacks and destroys brain cells. A variety of this reported recently in England is mad cow disease.

The degree of dementia depends upon the number of brain cells destroyed or damaged, and generally the condition is progressive. There is a normal age-related slow decrease in memory, known as benign senescent forgetfulness, from which everyone suffers to a greater or lesser degree as they age. This should not be confused with dementia, and you should not be frightened by occasional forgetfulness and believe that you are becoming demented. In dementia, the condition may start gradually, but it progresses as time goes on. In the early phases, items of daily use (keys, checkbook) may be misplaced. The person may have difficulty finding words to express herself and may forget details of daily activities and appointments. Later, more serious problems may arise. She may forget to turn off the oven or gas burners after cooking a meal. She may have difficulty balancing her checkbook, and finally she may become lost in her own neighborhood. Over time, she will gradually become disoriented and may not recognize her close relatives and friends.

Early detection can be helpful in slowing progression in some cases. If the problem is multiple infarcts of the brain due to hypertension, therapy may slow this process by restoring blood pressure to normal. Tacrine (cognex) is an example the new pharmacological agents that offer some hope in slowing the progression of Alzheimer's disease, and it is likely that more will be developed in the future. Dementia due to chronic alcoholism may be helped by stopping the use of alcohol, and currently medications being developed for the treatment of HIV infection offer some hope of prolonging the natural history of the disease, therefore putting off dementia for a period of time, at least. There is some recent data suggesting that estrogen may be helpful in slowing the process of dementia, particularly that related to Alzheimer's disease.

Even if it is not possible to slow the process of dementia, knowing that this is occurring may help families understand why a woman is demonstrating behavior changes and help them plan for her future. Supportive resources can be considered, such as home health care givers, who can help provide some of the twenty-four-hour-a-day coverage that may be necessary. Decisions regarding placing the patient in an assisted living or nursing home situation can also be considered.

DELIRIUM

While dementia is an organic problem, delirium is usually a physiologic problem. It is a disorder of brain physiology and often is reversible, but it is more commonly seen in older people. Table 17.3 lists the general causes of delerium.

In delirium, the brain experiences a global disruption of metabolic equilibrium. While it may occur in patients with dementia, it can certainly occur in those who have

TABLE 17.3. Delirium Disorders of Brain Physiology

Hypoxia (poor oxygenation)

Electrolyte imbalance

Hypoglycemia

Metabolic problems

External toxins (drugs)

Central nervous system infections

TABLE 17.4. Diagnostic Criteria for Delirium

1. Disturbance of consciousness with reduced ability to focus, sustain, or shift attention

2. A change in cognition, such as memory deficit, disorientation, language disturbance, or the development of a perceptual disturbance that is not better accounted for by a preexisting established or evolving dementia

3. Development of the disturbance over a short period of time (usually hours to days) and tends to fluctuate during the course of the day

4. Evidence from history, physical examination, or lab findings that the disturbance is caused by direct physiological consequences of a general medical condition

no other brain pathology. It generally begins with a sudden onset of mental status change, usually marked by disorientation, confusion, inability to remember new information, and varying levels of consciousness. These symptoms may vary over hours from near normal mental status to significant impairment of orientation. The person may appear sleepy, may hallucinate, and may lose sense of time. The diagnostic criteria for delirium are listed in Table 17.4.

Delirium is often seen in older people who undergo surgical procedures. They may suffer transient lack of oxygen, imbalance of their fluids or electrolytes, a decrease in the ability of their body to nourish their brain cells (hypoglycemia), and other metabolic problems that relate to the anesthesia or operation itself. Drug use in the form of anesthetics or painkilling agents may also affect brain function. Because of this, most physicians will give much smaller doses of medications that can affect the brain to older patients than to younger ones, since they detoxify these substances more slowly and usually excrete them from the body more slowly. Obviously, illnesses that affect the body's physiology can also cause delirium. Severe dehydrating conditions such as acute and chronic diarrhea can be a factor. Certainly patients who have an infection involving the brain or spinal cord can suffer delirium.

CASE STUDY

Tilly is eighty-two years old and had undergone an abdominal hysterectomy for cancer of the uterus. During the evening following surgery, she was restless, cried out several times, was incoherent to the nursing staff, and tried to get out of bed. Because of this, side rails were placed on her bed, and she was partially restrained. This led to further shouting, attempts to get out of bed, and incoherent speech. She was seen by a staff physician, who ordered a tranquilizer, and after this was administered, she fell into a deep sleep from which she did not awaken for eighteen hours. After she woke up, her brain function gradually became normal after she was given oxygen and her serum electrolytes were placed in balance. Her pain medications were decreased.

This is a typical example of an elderly patient's becoming delirious after the metabolic disruption of a surgical procedure. It was clearly not recognized by the staff taking care of her. She was instead treated with a tranquilizer, which put her into a deep sleep. Fortunately, her problem was recognized, and with oxygen, correction of her electrolyte balance, and time, she recovered. Most hospitals administer oxygen to elderly people in the postoperative period. The decrease in oxygen to their brain (hypoxia) is fairly common because of poor circulation. Their compensatory mechanisms for adjusting their fluid and electrolyte imbalance are also impaired because of age, and this needs to be watched very closely. Finally, medication must be used in very small amounts because of the difficulty that elderly patients have detoxifying and eliminating these.

CASE STUDY

Yvonne is a seventy-two-year-old woman who was diagnosed with inoperable kidney cancer, which had metastasized to bone by the time it was discovered. She was not yet terminal but was suffering from pain and was fearful. Her physician ordered appropriate pain medications but also added a moderate dose of the tranquilizer Valium. At first, she felt much better, but gradually she began to behave strangely. She believed that she was a young woman and was asking for her children, all of whom were grown and in distant cities. As time went on she became more agitated and had to be restrained. Her caregivers did not recognize that delirium was occurring, and her dose of Valium was increased. Finally, a physician was consulted, and Yvonne was admitted to the hospital, where the proper diagnosis was made. With supportive therapy and discontinuance of the Valium, her mental status slowly resolved.

Valium is a drug that is detoxified by the liver. In many older people it is detoxified slowly, leading to a building up of the medication within the system. This apparently happened with Yvonne, and since it was not recognized in its earlier form, the medication was increased rather than being stopped. Fortunately, the delirium was recognized early enough to be reversible.

CONCLUSIONS

Depression, dementia, and delirium are major issues in older people. It is helpful to recognize these in their earliest forms so that therapy can be offered. Women with depression can certainly be helped with medication and, at times, with psychiatric and social intervention. Women with dementia can often be helped if the condition can be recognized early and if appropriate treatment for the specific cause is available. Delirium should always be reversible if it is detected early enough. An older person behaving strangely or demonstrating a change in personality or behavior should be carefully evaluated. This is not normal behavior for the average older person, and the reason for the behavior change should be sought.

CHAPTER 18

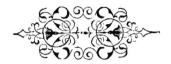

Facing Surgery:
What You Should Know and Expect

In the past, surgery has often been avoided as a therapeutic approach for older people because the risk of mortality was thought to be high and often not worth the effort. With improved pre- and postoperative care, better surgical techniques, and improvements in anesthesia, most elderly people can now undergo surgery safely and enjoy the benefits it has to offer. Surgical mortality is low in the elderly who are in good health or whose underlying medical problems are well controlled. Serious compromise of their heart, kidney, or lung status, however, increases their surgical risk, and it is important for a surgeon to understand the physiologic reserves of these various organ systems before submitting an older person to an operation. People with chronic illness or with unhealthy lifestyle patterns such as heavy smoking are at far greater risk in surgery than those who have compromised organ systems but are reasonably well controlled. Their problems not only may occur during the operation itself but also may lead to complications in the postoperative period.

INFORMED CONSENT

Physicians are ethically and legally bound to discuss a planned procedure with their patients, outlining alternative therapies that may be applied in the individual case as well as the risks that may be present if the procedure is carried out. Risks may involve potential injury to other organs, impairment of the function of the organ that will be operated upon, and the general risks of infection, hemorrhage, loss of function, or death. While for most procedures these risks are minimum, it is appropriate for a woman to know what they are so that she may weigh the potential benefits of having a procedure against the risks that she may incur. If an operation is suggested, ask a lot of questions. If your physician has not made clear to you why the operation is to be performed and what it will accomplish, ask for clarification. Do not be embarrassed or assume that you should know what your physician is implying. You should be perfectly clear about what will be undertaken. If risks are present, as they almost always are, you should understand clearly what they are and what the likelihood of complications may be. You should always ask if there are nonsurgical or other surgical approaches for solving your problem.

If an incision is to be made, its placement and size should be described for you. You should be told how long you can expect to be in the hospital and whether the procedure will be done as an inpatient, or what you will need to look for if you will be an outpatient and will go home after the procedure is completed. If it is important that you have someone stay with you after an operation, you should be made aware of this so that you may make these arrangements in advance. You should know how long you will be disabled and unable to work, and you should also be told when you will be able to resume your normal activities.

For each therapeutic approach that is offered, the potential benefits must be weighed against doing nothing or considering alternate therapy. Not every operation is necessary, and at times there are reasonable nonsurgical therapies that can be tried. It is best to leave your physician's office with clear information about the procedure, the risks involved, whether there are alternate therapies, the risks of doing nothing, how the operation will be performed, how long you will be disabled, when you will be able to expect a return to normal function, what permanent changes will be necessary in your life because of the procedure, and how you will be able to relate to others of significance in your life after the procedure has been performed. These are very individual questions, and the answers will not be the same for everyone. If you are not clear on these points, you should ask your physician for clarification. If it is not forthcoming, you should certainly seek a second opinion from another physician. Second opinions are always a good idea, particularly if the procedure being offered is a major one with strong ramifications for your life and well-being. Unless the procedure is being done as an emergency, you should take all the time you need to be sure you understand what will be undertaken.

Physicians are required to give complete information, including the risks involved, before obtaining a patient's informed consent. This can often frighten patients. They would rather hear that complications rarely occur and that the physician will do everything in his or her power to avoid them. Usually this is the case, but it is very important for patients to take an active role in their therapy and to be sure that they understand what risks, if any, are involved. It is necessary that this information be shared with you, even though you may feel quite overwhelmed and overburdened, making it difficult for you to consent to an operation that you really need and that may have very little risk associated with it. Also, most hospitals, in their attempt to satisfy informed consent rules, may end up having several people requesting your informed consent for various aspects of the operation. The anesthesiologist will discuss the risk of the anesthesia, the surgeon will discuss the risks of the surgery, the special care nurses may discuss the risks of the procedures for which they are responsible, and other therapists may also come by to discuss their part of your therapy and to describe any risks that may be associated with what they have to offer.

CASE STUDY

Gilda had a serious cancer and was hospitalized for a mastectomy and the subsequent placement of a central venous catheter through which she could then receive chemotherapy. She was also to receive postoperative irradiation therapy. Her surgeon first discussed her operation, and then the placement of the venous line. Next the anesthesiologist came by and discussed the risks of the anesthesia. Fortunately, they were considered to be minimal, and Gilda was able to process these into her thoughts appropriately. However, shortly after that, the nurse who was to be responsible for the care of the venous line came by and went over every possible complication that one could find with such a line. She talked about infection and the fact that the line might have to be removed or an antibiotic might have to be put into it. She talked about the risk of formation of clots on the line and the fact that they could move to other parts of the her body, causing complications, and finally she talked about the possibility of an air embolism. By this time, Gilda was extremely frightened. Since the line was to be in for several months, she asked the nurse what she should do if she had an air embolism. The nurse was perplexed, as she had never heard of one actually occurring, or seen one, and she suggested that Gilda had best call 911. At this point the anesthesiologist reentered the room, heard the conversation, and said a few words to put Gilda at ease. Shortly thereafter the radiology resident entered the room to discuss the radiation Gilda would need to have. Again, a list of very unlikely serious complications was presented to her. By this time, she was seriously considering leaving the hospital. Clearly, she had been the victim of too much information.

Most hospitals will allow one person to give each patient all of the information needed for informed consent. This usually is the physician primarily responsible for the care of the patient, and only this physician delegates certain aspects of the care to others involved. There are always risks for procedures, but their magnitude may be quite variable. The patient cannot be expected to understand these without explanation, so if you are in this situation, you should ask specific questions so that you understand exactly what risks you are facing.

PREOPERATIVE ASSESSMENT

No patients should face surgery without an adequate preoperative assessment of their physical status. This is particularly true for older people. The American Society of Anesthesiologists has developed a classification of patients' physical status in order to assess the risks of general anesthesia and postoperative complications. Such a classification gives the surgeon and the anesthesiologist some idea of the patient's surgical risk and alerts them to potential problems. (See Table 18.1.)

In general, studies have shown that patients classified as I and II do not tend to have cardiorespiratory problems when undergoing general surgical procedures.

TABLE 18.1.   Physical Status Classification of the American
Society of Anesthesiologists

Class	Definitions
I	Healthy patient
II	Mild systemic disease no functional limitations
III	Severe systemic disease with functional limitations
IV	Incapacitated patient
V	Moribund patient; not expected to survive 24 hours with or without surgery

Patients who are status III or above are identified as at high risk and usually require additional studies to determine specific risks. Most of the elderly fall into the II and III risk categories, making it important that surgeons identify their risks preoperatively and take whatever steps they can to correct other medical problems before the surgery is carried out.

In order to obtain the information the surgeon needs to make specific judgments, a careful general health history and complete physical examination should be carried out. Surgeons usually obtain a history of previous surgical procedures by getting operative reports from previous surgeons so that they may note what has been done in the past and whether or not complications were suffered. Surgeons generally do not rely on patient's memory alone. A family history is also important because it allows the surgeon to see trends such as cancer-prone families, chronic illnesses that may run in families, sensitivities to medications, or allergies.

Appropriate lab studies should be obtained, depending upon the proposed operation and the patient's general health. Certainly, cardiac, pulmonary, and kidney status should be evaluated. Also, mental status should be evaluated so that precautions can be taken to preserve this postoperatively and to avoid delirium.

It is always important for a surgeon to understand the patient's problem completely and to have a good grasp of the patient's physical condition before proceeding to surgery. It is also important that the surgeon make sure that the patient understands the necessity and the consequences of the surgery before proceeding. Unless there is a need for emergency treatment, the assessment of the patient and the development of an understanding between the patient and the physician about the need for the surgery and how it will be performed should be done over time. It is probably not a good idea to decide upon a surgical procedure on the first visit to the surgeon and then proceed immediately. The patient should have a positive attitude toward the surgery.

In emergency situations, these suggestions often must be modified. However, it is important that as many aspects of informed consent and preoperative evaluation be carried out as possible so that the patient may undergo surgery with the best possible circumstances.

CHOICE OF ANESTHESIA

Most people wish to discuss with the surgeon the anesthesia that will be used at the time that the operation is planned. It is best to include the anesthesiologist in this discussion. In most settings, this is done at a separate time. I usually tell a patient the type of anesthesia that will be appropriate in the procedure contemplated based on her age, general medical condition, and the task that is to be physically performed. I suggest that she discuss these possibilities with the anesthesiologist who will have the responsibility for her well-being at the time of the operation.

Three types of anesthesia can be applied. The first is local anesthesia, in which the area to be incised is infiltrated with a local anesthetic such as xylocaine or novacaine. There are many agents available, and each has its advantages and disadvantages. Local anesthesia is adequate for many biopsies or minor procedures. It can also be applied in fairly major procedures if the patient is cooperative. Since local anesthesia carries minimal risk, it is often appropriate for use in high-risk patients whose cardiac, pulmonary, or general health status may be such that a general or other regional anesthetic may create a serious risk to their well-being. I have performed many pelvic reparative procedures in very elderly women who were under local anesthesia.

The second type of anesthesia is regional anesthesia. Many anesthetic approaches fall under this category. These include nerve blocks, which are extremely useful for surgery on hands or limbs, and epidural anesthesia, in which a local anesthetic agent is placed into the epidural space surrounding the nerves as they come from the spinal cord. This type of anesthetic differs from a spinal anesthetic in that the spinal fluid is not entered and the anesthetic is rather diffused around the nerve roots after they have left the spinal fluid. It is an excellent anesthesia for abdominal and pelvic procedures. A third type of regional anesthesia is a spinal block. The anesthesia is placed directly into the spinal fluid. This also is a very effective anesthesia for pelvic and abdominal surgery. The advantage of regional anesthesia is that the patient may be kept awake or lightly sedated, thereby preventing the risk of pulmonary complications that may be present with general anesthesia. These methods will give good anesthesia, and generally if an epidural anesthesia is being used, it can be continued in small doses after the operation for pain relief. Patients who have regional anesthesia usually are responsive more rapidly and tend to be less nauseated and groggy after the operation is performed than women who have had a general anesthesia. The anesthetic that is chosen depends upon the skills of the anesthesiologist, the anatomy of the patient, and whether or not the patient desires to be awake during the procedure. For gynecologic operations, epidural or spinal anesthesia is an excellent choice.

The third type of anesthetic available is a general anesthetic. In this situation, the patient is put to sleep using either gases, injectable anesthetics, or a combination of both. With these methods, the anesthesiologist can sedate the patient lightly or deeply, depending upon the need of the operation. Thus, general anesthetics are generally given in conjunction with a substance used to paralyze the muscles so that good relaxation can be obtained for the surgical procedure. Most anesthesiologists are very adept at using these various agents and will choose the appropriate one for the patient's risk factors and general condition.

For any given case, the anesthesiologist may suggest the specific anesthetic that is deemed safest for that particular circumstance. If a choice exists, the anesthesiologist will generally discuss this with the patient, and they will come to a decision jointly. Occasionally the surgeon will have a strong feeling about the anesthetic that would be best and will relate this to the patient and the anesthesiologist for their consideration. The bottom line is that the choice of anesthesia should be individualized for each patient and her circumstances, and she should be able to choose if possible.

POTENTIAL COMPLICATIONS

Complications of surgery in modern times are quite uncommon. Nevertheless, they do occur, and physicians will take steps to try to prevent them. Some problems, however, are not preventable, and the physician will make every effort to try to recognize them early and treat them if necessary. Even minor complications may lead to more serious problems if they are not dealt with.

In the immediate postoperative period, the hospital staff will be vigilant for signs of blood loss and heart, lung, or kidney problems. Depending upon the type of operation, the blood loss may be internal or external, and patients are monitored with respect to pulse and blood pressure. In general, rapid pulse may imply blood loss, as will dropping blood pressure. Therefore, if you have had a major operation, your pulse and blood pressure will be monitored at very frequent intervals throughout the first twelve to twenty-four postoperative hours. If the pulse is found to be becoming rapid or blood pressure is dropping, your physician will generally order a hematocrit in order to determine whether or not you are becoming anemic. Pulse and blood pressure changes may be related to your anesthetic and the reestablishment of your normal physiologic state and may not necessarily mean blood loss. It will be up to your physician to evaluate you further to determine which is the case. If you have had a long operation with a fairly significant blood loss and have not had a blood transfusion, your physician will probably first try to replace your lost fluid volume with crystalloid solutions while monitoring your hematocrit and general well-being. Older women cannot tolerate a major degree of anemia, as it may lead to coronary artery insufficiency. The heart muscle requires blood for oxygenation, and if the coronary arteries are already partially compromised, blood of a low hematocrit may not deliver enough oxygen to the heart muscles to satisfy their needs. In such a situation, blood may be important. As you were prepared for surgery, you may have been asked to bank your own blood (autologous blood). If there is enough time prior to surgery and your condition is favorable, it may have been possible to put either one or two units of blood into the blood bank for you. If this is the case, the physician will probably be quite liberal in returning it to you. If you have none or not enough autologous blood available, you may require a blood transfusion from a donor. In this day and age, most physicians try very hard not to replace blood unless it is absolutely necessary. On the other hand, it may be life-saving and necessary. Most people fear contracting HIV with a blood transfusion. Actually, that is quite rare, as blood banks screen effectively for this. The risk of certain types of hepatitis in blood bank blood is real, however, although screening for these is also being utilized. A good rule of thumb followed by most physicians, which is reasonable for the patient to keep in mind, is that blood should not be given unless it is absolutely needed. If it is needed, the benefits probably far outweigh the risks that may exist.

Occasionally a patient may be found to be bleeding excessively, usually due to the fact that a ligature has slipped. In such instances, the patient will be returned to the operating room to control the bleeding. This is a rare event, but under such circumstances it could be life-saving.

Older patients are at risk for coronary artery insufficiency, particularly if they have had excessive blood loss, and they should be monitored for cardiac function in the immediate postoperative period. If they are placed in the intensive care unit, as they often are for short periods of time, their electrocardiogram is continuously monitored. Evidence of cardiac muscle ischemia (lack of oxygen) therefore is usually picked up rapidly, allowing treatment to be started. In the elderly not only may the coronary arteries be insufficient, but so may the arterial system to the brain. In order to help protect both the brain and the heart, it is fairly customary to administer oxygen, usually through a nasal catheter to older individuals, during the immediate postoperative period.

The patient's lung function is also extremely important, because this is where oxygen is exchanged with the blood and carbon dioxide and other waste products are removed. Often in the immediate postoperative period, particularly if the patient has had a long operative procedure and a general anesthetic, the lungs do not inflate adequately, decreasing their ability to exchange oxygen and waste products. Therefore, in the immediate postoperative period, patients are encouraged to breathe deeply and cough, to bring up mucus that may be collected in the bronchial tree and to help open up the air pockets within the lungs (alveoli). This is referred to as pulmonary toilet, and hospital personnel will encourage patients in this activity, at least during the first twenty-four to forty-eight hours. Smokers are often more greatly affected by the problem of mucus in the pulmonary tree than are nonsmokers, but smokers often cough better and may clear the problem more rapidly than do nonsmokers. Older people who have more rigid bronchial trees need particular encouragement to carry out their pulmonary toilet.

Occasionally, particularly in patients who have had a general anesthetic, aspiration of stomach contents into the bronchial tree may take place. This usually occurs at the time the patient is being awakened from the anesthetic and is one of the reasons anesthesiologists often feel safer to place an endotracheal tube into the patient's trachea for the surgical procedure. The stomach contents are quite acidic, and this is very irritating to the lungs. Aspiration pneumonia may develop. Usually it is mild, but it can be quite serious, so physicians will monitor their patient's pulmonary function by listening to the chest frequently and by being sure that both lungs are entirely aerated.

The final organ system that is monitored in the immediate postoperative period is the kidneys. Patients will often put out very little urine immediately after surgery. This may be because of the shock of the operation to the body or because they have not had sufficient fluids during the procedure. Generally, within the first few hours after surgery, the patient begins to make adequate amounts of urine, and this can be measured and monitored. Often, if the fluid output is minimal, more intravenous fluids will be given.

Bowel function usually returns within a few days after an abdominal procedure. At first bowel tones can be heard; next the patient will pass gas, and finally she will have a bowel movement. Occasionally, bowel sounds do not return rapidly, and the bowel may become distended with gas. Often this is transient, but rarely the process continues for a longer period of time. This complication is called adynamic ileus and is essentially a quiet bowel. It is treated by not feeding the patient by mouth but rather continuing intravenous feedings. Occasionally a nasogastric suction tube will be placed through the nose into the stomach to help decompress the gas. Oral feeding is not begun until bowel sounds return.

Fortunately adynamic ileus rarely occurs, and most patients will begin oral feedings as soon as bowel sounds are noted (via the stethoscope) by the physician.

A later but serious complication of an operation may be infection. Generally, infection does not occur during the first postoperative day and frequently does not show up until the second day. Infection may be in the wound, in the lungs in the form of pneumonia, or in the bladder due to a Foley catheter's having been placed during the operation. In rare instances, the bladder infection may rise up the urinary tract and cause a kidney infection (pyelitis). The first sign of infection is usually fever, and fevers in excess of 100.4°F are generally considered significant. If a patient runs a fever on the second postoperative day, the physician will generally investigate the urine, the lungs, and the wound. Wound infections are quite uncommon but do occur following prolonged surgery or surgery that is contaminated, such as opening a loop of colon. Bladder infections are very common, particularly in older people who may have bacteria in their urine to start with. Kidney infections are much less common and usually occur only after a bladder infection has been present for a while. Lung infections (pneumonia) occur but are most often due to aspiration in the postoperative period.

When infection occurs, the area involved should be cultured and specific antibiotics begun. Fever during the first postoperative day is quite common and is usually due to the inability of the lungs to completely inflate (atelectasis). The appropriate management of this is to take steps to increase aeration of the lungs.

A later postoperative complication may be thrombophlebitis in the extremities, that is, the clotting of blood within the veins of the legs. It is seen frequently following orthopedic surgery involving the lower extremities and after prolonged abdominal surgery. Surgeons generally attempt to prevent this by applying pneumatic appliances to the legs which continue the circulation of blood while the patient is anesthetized and into the postoperative period, or with other means such as elastic stockings used during and after the procedure. In patients considered to be at high risk, blood thinning medications such as heparin are also used in small doses. If heparin is used, the benefits must be weighed against the risk of hemorrhage that may occur during the procedure because of the modification of the clotting mechanism. Patients with cancer seem to be at greater risk than others of developing thrombophlebitis. Generally, surgeons performing cancer operations take the strongest precautions to prevent thrombophlebitis.

Thrombophlebitis is associated with a swollen, tender, usually warm leg, but the real risk is that a piece of the clot may break lose and migrate to the lungs, causing a pulmonary embolism. If the embolism is large enough it may cause acute collapse of the pulmonary and circulatory systems and may lead to death. If it is a small embolism it will probably affect only a small portion of the lung and will be noted as chest pain, cough, and sometimes coughing up blood. When such symptoms occur in the postoperative period, physicians will generally evaluate the patient rapidly to determine if this is what has happened. The treatment for pulmonary embolism and thrombophlebitis is anticoagulation, using medications such as heparin.

The final complication of the postoperative period is the disruption of the wound. Most of the time it is superficial and is caused by an infection in the fat and subcutaneous tissue. In this situation, there is frequently a buildup of pus beneath the skin, causing an opening of the skin incision and the release of the pus. Generally, if this is all that is present, the patient rapidly gets better, and the wound heals in. On the other hand, if the fascia beneath the subcutaneous tissue breaks down, the entire wound may open. This is called a dehiscence, and it is considered an emergency situation. The patient is taken to the operating room, where the wound is cleaned (debrided) and then closed. Often in such situations the skin is left open to reduce the chance of wound infection recurring. Actually, this is a very rare complication in most surgical procedures.

In modern times, these major postoperative complications are fortunately quite rare. Your physician should discuss these possibilities in light of any procedure that you may be contemplating, so that you may keep a proper prospective.

AFTER YOU GO HOME

When you go home depends upon the type of procedure that you have had. If you have had an outpatient procedure, you will probably be home in a matter of hours. If you have had a major operative procedure in the hospital, you will be sent home in a matter of days or weeks, depending upon the severity of the condition and your postoperative course. Generally, if the procedure is relatively minor, you will probably return to normal activities almost immediately, modifying your behavior only to allow your wound to heal. If, on the other hand, you have had a major procedure with an anesthetic, although you may feel perfectly normal in a very short period of time, your reflexes, hand-eye coordination, and ability to react to emergency situations such as might occur if you were driving a car or working on a piece of equipment may not come completely back for 3–4 weeks. I usually advise patients not to drive cars or run major pieces of equipment for at least 3–4 weeks after an operation.

Second, your stamina and endurance will be reduced after a surgical procedure. Therefore, activities that you normally enjoy should be modified. If you like to walk for exercise, you probably can begin to do this a few weeks after a major operation but the distance you try to travel and the speed at which you go should be modified to meet your available energy. At no time should you push yourself beyond what your body tells you it can handle. To do so, will probably cause your wound to hurt for a longer period than necessary and you may sense that you are not getting your energy back as quickly as you would like.

Wounds heal by the development of collagen across the cut surfaces. The tensile strength of a wound is probably at its weakest 4–5 days after the procedure but quickly improves thereafter. Generally, by about 3 months the wound is 90% healed. Depending upon the type of procedure you have had, you should keep this in mind as you increase the activities in which you normally participate. You will probably feel reasonably good by about 3 months after a major operation but it may take 9 months to a year to get back to a completely normal state. You should be patient with yourself and not expect more of your body than it can handle. On the other hand, it is important to begin modified activities as soon after the operation as you can in order to return your muscle tone, your energy level, and your stamina, as soon as possible. Your doctor will give you guidelines to follow and you should feel comfortable performing within those guidelines.

Summary

It is best to be sure when an operation is contemplated that it is absolutely necessary and that you understand all of the alternatives of therapy. It is equally important to clearly understand what will be done, how it will be done, and what condition you will be in when the surgery is completed. It is important to integrate the significant people in your life into this experience. If there are any questions, a second opinion should always be obtained.

You should enter a surgical experience in the best of health, condition and the best frame of mind possible. This will be aided by your understanding what is about to happen. If your operation has a good chance of being associated with significant blood loss and you can donate your blood for your own use ahead of time, you should do so. Getting family members to contribute blood is important for the overall function of your blood bank, but it will not necessarily help you. It has been shown that even family members with the same blood type offer about the same amount of risk for infection as does the general population.

Postoperatively you should work diligently with your hospital staff to help your recovery. If they encourage you to address your pulmonary toilet, you should do so to the best of your ability. You will probably be asked to move about as soon as possible after surgery, and you will be given fluids and solid foods as soon as your GI tract can tolerate them.

It is very fashionable today, because of the high cost of medical care, to discharge people from the hospital as soon as possible. This is not necessarily bad; most patients who are beyond any dangerous period of their postoperative course are more comfortable at home. You should be sure that you have someone readily available to help you in case some unexpected emergency occurs.

In the postoperative period, you may work to get your strength and stamina back by engaging in the activities in which you normally participate. These should be done with moderation and common sense, and only those that pose no danger should be utilized in the postoperative period. Following these relatively simple steps should enable you to go through your surgery in the best possible physical and psychological state.

INDEX

Cancer (*continued*)
  colorectal, 96–98
  death rates, 93–94
  endometrial, 45–46, 104–105
  lung, 95
  ovarian (*See* Ovarian cancer)
  vaginal, 101
  vulvar, 99–101
Candida albicans, 123
Carbohydrates, 21, 23–24
Cardiac output, 32
Cardinal ligaments, 142
Cardiovascular disease, 49, 89–91
CASS (Coronary Artery Surgery
  Study), 90
Cerebral vascular disease (stroke), 50,
  90, 91
Cervical cancer, 101–103, 126
Chemotherapy, for breast cancer, 83
Child, death of, 153–154
Cholesterol, serum
  estrogen and, 23, 49–50, 90
  screening, 15
Chromium, 27
Chronic illnesses, nutrition and, 19
Cigarette smoking, cessation of, 5
Cimetidine, 42
Clear cell carcinoma, of vagina, 101
Climara, 53
Clonidine, 56
Coccygeus, 141
Cognex (tacrine), 170
Collagen, 49, 132
Colonoscopy, 97
Colorectal cancer, 96–98
Colpocleisis, 150
Colporrhaphy
  anterior, 134, 145, 150
  posterior, 147, 150
Compazine, 129
Complaint, chief, 9
Complications, postoperative, 180–
  183
Conjugated equine estrogens
  (Premarin), 52–53
Continence, 127–130

Coronary artery disease, 33, 35,
  89–91
Coronary artery insufficiency, 180, 181
Coronary Artery Surgery Study
  (CASS), 90
Corticosteroids, 121
Coumadin, 43
Creutzfeldt-Jakob disease, 170
Cystadenocarcinomas, 106–107
Cystadenoma, benign serous, 114
Cystic tumors, ovarian, 113
Cystocele, 134, 142–146
Cysts
  mammographic detection of, 81
  ovarian, 112–113

D

D&C (dilation and curettage), 104, 105
Death
  from cancer, 93–94
  impending, 160–161
Dehiscence, 183
Delirium, 163, 170–173
Dementia, 163, 169–170
Denial, of impending death, 160
Depo Provera, 47
Depression
  agitated, 157–158
  bereavement and, 164–166
  diagnosis of, 166–167
  eating habits and, 19
  estrogen and, 57–59
  exercises for, 33, 35, 36
  major, 166–167
  minor, 165
  over impending death, 161
  suicidal ideation and, 167
  treatment, 167–169
Dermatoses, vulvar, 122
DES (diethylstilbestrol), 13–14, 101
Desyrel (trazadone), 168
Diabetes mellitus
  exercises for, 33, 35

Hypoxia, 172
Hysterectomy, 103, 105, 106

I

Ileus, adynamic, 182
Imidazoles, 123
Imipramine, 137
Immune system dysfunction, exercises
    for, 33, 35
Immunizations
    contraindications for, 64
    for high-risk situations, 62–64
    for older women, 16–17
    recommendations for, 61–62, 65
    record of, 11
    routine, 61–62
    for travel, 62, 63, 64, 65
Incontinence
    bladder instability-urge, 136–138
    evaluation of, 130–132
    exercises for, 33, 35
    incentive, 138
    incidence, 10, 127
    overflow, 138
    treatment of, 132–136
Infections
    bladder, 138–139
    postoperative, 182
Influenza vaccine, 16, 61–62
Informed consent, 175–177
Intraocular pressure, 12
Intrinsic sphincter deficiency (ISD),
    135–136
Iodine, 25
Iron, 25, 26, 27
Ischiocavernosus muscle, 142
ISD (intrinsic sphincter deficiency),
    135–136
Isoxsuprine, 129

J

Job, loss of, 159–160

K

Kegel exercises, 130, 133
Kidneys
    aging process and, 23, 40
    postoperative monitoring,
        181–182
Kraurosis, 121

L

Laboratory tests, screening, 14–16
LDL (low-density lipoprotein),
    49–50, 87
Leiomyomas. *See* Fibroids
Leiomyosarcoma, 112
Leukemia, 108–109
Levator ani muscles, 141
Levodopa, 28, 129
LH (luteinizing hormone), 47–48
Libido, loss of, 73–74
Lichen sclerosis, 99, 121
Lipids, dietary recommendations,
    23
Liver
    aging process and, 40
    disease, hormone replacement
        and, 56
Local anesthesia, 179
Loss
    of child, 153–154
    depression and, 164–166
    grief reaction from (*See* Grief)
    of job, 159–160
    of organ or body part, 158
    of pet, 159
    of spouse, 154
Low-density lipoprotein (LDL), 49–50,
    87
Lumpectomy, 83
Lung cancer, 95
Lung function, postoperative, 181
Luteinizing hormone (LH), 47–48
Lymphomas, 108